Advance Praise

"Leah Carver offers a refreshing, empowering approach to wellness in *Undoing Hashimoto's*. Her creative insights provide hope not only for those of us with autoimmune disorders, but for all women seeking a journey toward self-care. *Undoing* is the most transformative book I have read in some time. I felt the author was speaking directly to me in a calm, nonjudgmental, understanding way. The beauty of the book is also in its simplicity. Carver advocates for slow, small, gradual change while recognizing the reader could easily feel overwhelmed by the many layers of transformation that may needed. During my first read of *Undoing*, I became acutely aware of my "burnt toast syndrome" and began to introduce wellness techniques such as spending time in nature, exploring the benefits of water, and experimenting with hot and cold. I look forward to deepening my own wellness practice and look forward to sharing this book with family, friends, and patients."

– HOLLY LaSALLE-RICCI, PHD

"Leah Carver's *Undoing Hashimoto's* struck my core. I do not have Hashimoto's and yet, I felt every word spoke to me. Well-written, clear, and with compassion, Carver's words touched every part of my life ... my marriage, my children, my professional life, my spiritual journey as a whole. I have implemented many of the simple practices and been reminded of my power and worth. I am grateful for this book and feel it is valuable for all people, regardless of the path."

– LANI SCOZZARI, MFA

Undoing Hashimoto's

un**doing**
HASHIMOTO'S

A Guide to Managing Symptoms,
Relieving Overwhelm, and Living Well

LEAH CARVER

NEW YORK

LONDON • NASHVILLE • MELBOURNE • VANCOUVER

undoing HASHIMOTO'S

A Guide to Managing Symptoms, Relieving Overwhelm
and Living Well

Published in New York, New York, by Morgan James Publishing in partnership with Difference Press. Morgan James is a trademark of Morgan James, LLC. www.MorganJamesPublishing.com

The Morgan James Speakers Group can bring authors to your live event. For more information or to book an event visit The Morgan James Speakers Group at www.TheMorganJamesSpeakersGroup.com.

ISBN 9781683509394 paperback
ISBN 9781683509400 eBook
Library of Congress Control Number: 2018930954

Cover Design by:
Christopher Kirk
www.GFSstudio.com

Interior Design by:
Chris Treccani
www.3dogcreative.net

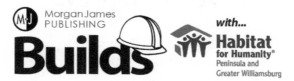

In an effort to support local communities, raise awareness and funds, Morgan James Publishing donates a percentage of all book sales for the life of each book to Habitat for Humanity Peninsula and Greater Williamsburg.

Get involved today! Visit
www.MorganJamesBuilds.com

For my many teachers, all shapes and sizes.

Table of Contents

Introduction

*"Maybe who we are isn't so much about what
we do, but rather what we're capable of when
we least expect it."*
JODI PICOULT

I know you have been researching all the right things to do since you got your diagnosis of Hashimoto's Thyroiditis. Maybe you have even tried to go on the Auto-Immune Paleo Diet or some other form of an elimination/anti-inflammatory diet, but things came up: a birthday party or holiday. Maybe you just don't feel good and feel like you need sugar to get you through the day. But you know you can't stay where you are, or things won't get better. You know the only way to make the pain better is to try something different, but you don't know where to start and you don't want to fail again.

It is not easy to hold yourself accountable and make changes when you don't feel well. You may be struggling with brain fog, fatigue, physical pain, headaches, depression, and so much more. When you look to Facebook groups, some people seem to have had no problem making the lifestyle changes they needed and yet here you are, struggling to understand or even remember what you just read you were supposed to do. How come it seems easy for some people and almost impossible for you? Why don't you have the willpower to make these necessary changes?

I spent lots of time ruminating on the answers to these questions. I discovered that it wasn't something I needed to push myself to create, in fact, it was the opposite. It was not more self-discipline, it was pulling back, looking inward, and reassessing the foundations I had built.

Stop putting unrealistic expectations on yourself and then having to deal with the feeling of failure or anger or shame when you fail. It's time to shift the way you look at the problem. Don't waste important energy blaming yourself for getting sick or thinking that somehow you deserve this. In general, life is a figure-it-out-as-you-go kind of thing. You may have a master's degree in business or education, for example, but it doesn't mean you should be able to navigate all of life's twists and turns alone. Instead, know that you are going to struggle and that there is no place of unchanging perfection. Allow the struggle, but work to build resiliency and stability. This is the key question: How can we set ourselves up for success? Right now, what you know is that you are not feeling well, and you're probably exhausted and just wishing for a miracle. If you can just put your trust in me for a little while, know that I have been there in the struggle just like you, completely exhausted, and with not much left to give. I know how to start shifting the way you are feeling, because I did it for myself and for many others. Let me help the tired, overwhelmed you navigate this part of the journey. Of course you wish this was not your situation, but it is, and now you will have the tools to transform. Right now, you may be wishing everything could just go back to how it was before the pain, and while that is not something I can guarantee, my hope for you is that you will grow profoundly. If you integrate these steps into your life, you will begin to once again feel inspired and excited about life.

In this book, I will present to you some information that changed the game for me. I'll introduce you to tools that will awaken the power within you and help you feel a renewed sense of purpose in life.

I know there is a part of you right now that understands how important it is for you to make these changes. After all, here you are, reading another book in the hopes of gaining some more awareness and information on how to get well. How to respond on the days you feel pain, what to do when you are exhausted, and what you can take a chance on doing on the days when you feel pretty darn great. With autoimmune disease, you basically have two choices: suffer and continually see your symptoms get worse, or chose to engage and show up in a way that feels powerful and true. The latter way, there may still be days of pain, but not so much suffering.

I wrote this book for you; it is intended to help you reexamine and rebuild your foundation, a foundation on which to build your journey to wellness. What does it mean to reexamine your foundation? It means learning to access your soul, to begin to listen to your heart, to hear the underlying thoughts that have been driving your life, and begin to choose the big Yes over the little yes. To support your body as a means to build your power and create the life you want. Many books on the subject of Hashimoto's are rich with information, but can be overwhelming and difficult to understand when you feel your worst. I want you to know you are not alone; there are a lot of people, including myself, who have been right where you are now. I have a shelf full of books on Hashimoto's, and yet when I was at my sickest, all they seemed to do was reinforce my overwhelm. It was my experience that until I implemented the steps I'll take you through in this book, I consistently just strengthened the voice that was saying I wasn't capable or good enough. These steps made it possible for me to shift my lifestyle habits without feeling deprived or alienated. This process adds a softness that is necessary for you to make lasting changes, and have a sense of ease about them. I would argue that without the information in this book, you may struggle to enforce rules on yourself and chide yourself when you fail.

It is not about being perfect. In fact, it is about being gentle and kind. It's about setting realistic expectations of yourself and slowing down enough to notice your stuff. Pema Chodron says that "the most fundamental aggression to ourselves, the most fundamental harm we can do ourselves, is to remain ignorant by not having the courage and respect to look at ourselves honestly and gently."

This living and living well is not something most of us have been taught. We have to figure it out, and yet we have a perceived belief that we should know how to do everything already. When babies first learn to walk, they fall multiple times, but we don't chastise them, we encourage them to keep trying. At what point do we begin to set unrealistic expectations for ourselves and then tell ourselves we are not capable or not smart enough, etc.? Instead, if we show ourselves kindness and compassion on our journey to wellness, we will evolve into something beautiful.

It doesn't have to be hard. This is why I wrote this book. I had been in the spa and wellness industry for almost 20 years when I got my diagnosis of Hashimoto's Thyroiditis. Once you get a diagnosis – or even before – if instead of hurrying to fix it you just begin by following the method in this book, you will be able to gently and easily make lifestyle changes you desire, and stick with them.

If you don't know much about nutrition and the holistic health field, working on your own to make these changes can take a lot of time and energy. If instead you take the time to listen to your body, to soften to it and to learn how to nurture yourself, you will begin to build the energy you need to implement some of the more difficult or foreign concepts.

The following chapters are full of information and insights that will help you on your road to wellness. I recommend just reading it straight through, cover to cover, first. It is very intentionally easy reading because I understand right now you may not be up for a textbook. Don't worry about implementing all the exercises; just read the book. After you have finished the whole book and have an understanding of the path ahead, go back and re-read Chapters 2 through 7, giving yourself a week to practice the actions in each chapter before you move on.

The program is designed to be done in 6 weeks, so if you spend a week on each chapter, by the end you will have built your capacity to take in more information, to know which practices work best for you, and to understand how you can actively engage with what you are feeling in order to feel better.

This book will change your life in a positive way, and it will build your power to a place where making the next steps will come easily. The ideas in this book will serve you throughout your life as tool for creating the best possible life for you.

Use this book as an interactive guide – make notes in the margins or grab a companion journal. Write down ideas or questions that come up for you as you read. Think about ways that this applies to your life; where you can see alignment and where you feel stuck. Make it as applicable to you as possible, and as you read the stories, think about how they are similar to what you are going through.

I know you can evolve your relationship with your Hashimoto's autoimmune condition and begin to see it as a call to action. The great thing about this is that it is totally up to you. Keep this book next to your bed even after you have moved forward in the process. It will continue to work with and for you, building your awareness and capacity for growth.

Continue to do this work so that you can not only make these changes for yourself, but also so you can support and love the people closest to you in a powerful way. In this book, I will teach you the techniques for increasing energy and relaxation that I use not just with my clients, but with my children, for myself, and with the people closest to me.

The formula I have for developing the willpower you need to make these changes in your life is unique. Let me explain how.

I have practiced body work and spa therapies for years, and while they can be incredibly helpful, I found that people were looking to me not just to make them feel better, but to actually *become* better. In fact, they would often call me a healer. While I have absolutely no problem with healers, it was not what I wanted to do. I consider myself a facilitator. I want to give the power back to *you*. You see, I can teach you and help you develop the ability to take care of yourself. Not only do I find this more efficient, but I think it is even more empowering. If I teach you how to listen to your body and how to engage effectively with what you are feeling, then it doesn't matter whether it's 3:00 am and I am in Japan: You have the tools needed to take care of yourself.

Understanding that you are a physical body, an emotional body, an energy body, and a spiritual body is vital to your healing process. If you learn how to take care of all layers of you, then you will support true and lasting change. If, however, you compartmentalize and only treat one aspect of yourself, you will continue to struggle.

I had a client, Cindy, who for years had struggled to make any big changes in her life. When I asked her about her difficulty making the positive changes she'd said she wanted to make, she had a million excuses – and some of them were really quite good. I had her start my 6-step program, and before long she was making changes that didn't feel difficult for her. After week 5, she signed up to begin exercise classes and was actually enjoying it. She felt different and stronger, no longer so fragile. Something she had not been able to make herself do in the past because she was so exhausted, she could now do without any prompting. She just felt better.

I know you can do this. This process has worked for me and for many others before you, and it will work for you. Trust the process, and remember to be kind to yourself.

Chapter 1

The Reckoning

"We have to be brave enough to reckon with our deepest emotions."
BRENÉ BROWN

A few years ago, I was teaching yoga at my studio when I got a terrible virus known as CMV. I had a high fever, and my throat was incredibly sore. I was in the middle of teaching a training over the weekend, and after that I was leaving to go on vacation with my family for a week in the Florida Keys. I had been going at full throttle for the last four-plus years, and didn't see change in sight. I ate relatively well, though I will confess I was a closet sugar addict. Some days, it was the only thing that kept me going.

I have no idea why I showed up for work that weekend: I had other teachers who could have covered for me. There was just this part of me that thought I couldn't let people down. I worried about having to ask for help. Honestly, I was proud of my strength. I didn't need anyone. I think it was halfway through teaching that morning when I realized I had absolutely no idea what I was talking about. Sweat was dripping down my back (which was very unusual for me because I would never sweat). I realized I was not well! I left early and went home to pack for my trip. I laugh now in reflection. What was I thinking?

Thus began my reckoning. While we were in the Keys, I went out paddle boarding. I still had a high fever, but I didn't want to put a damper on the family vacation. I had my youngest on the front of my paddle board, and my husband was on another board with my eldest daughter. On the way back to the resort, the current shifted, and we now had to paddle against it. There was no paddling slowly; my husband had to paddle hard to make it under a bridge. He couldn't help me at all. I remember being on the board with the ocean pulling at me and thinking *I really don't know if I can do this, I don't think I have the strength it will take.* I dug deep, but there really wasn't much to give. I saw some jet skiers off in the distance and thought about flagging them down for help. It was about the most pitiful I have ever felt. We were only about 50 feet from the bridge when my little one said, "Mommy, I don't think we are getting anywhere."

This echoed an inner feeling in my life. I had been pushing and not listening for a long time by then. As much as I loved my job and my studio, I was beginning to realize I could not sustain the pace and life I was living. Even with jet skiers relatively close by who could save me, I didn't dare ask for help. I didn't want anyone to know how weak I was. There was a sense of shame and denial. If I could just manage to keep pushing a little bit more, then maybe everything would miraculously get better. I always told myself I didn't have a right to complain when there were so many others who had it worse than me. If I continued to pretend everything was ok, and everyone around me played their part, then we could continue on, but to what end?

I realized that no matter how hard I was trying, I didn't feel like I was getting anywhere. In fact, I commonly referred to life as "the hamster wheel." I felt like I was caught in the eternal spin, and the only relief came in the form of sleep, so of course I found myself just wanting to go to bed. In this moment, I was clearly able to see in my weakness and exhaustion that my habit of pushing harder was not serving me. I had to change, and I had to do it now.

Surrender was not a new concept to me; I had been taught about it in yoga. I thought I had done it, but just like most things, there are always layers, and so what felt like surrender was me actually pretending to surrender by being passive.

I was stuck in a place of not knowing how to stop. But this day, on the water, was the day I made a promise to myself to change. My physical and emotional strength had always worked for me, I thought, but as I began to look at how I got to that point, I realized it was just as much my weakness. As I reflect on it now, I can see how this infused all aspects of my life. I loved that I could show up in a stressful situation and manage it, solve problems, and fix things. The trouble with this was that time and time again, I would throw myself in at the deep end, believing I thrived on stress. As a "doer," or Type A, I had a belief that this was the time when I was most needed and loved.

People liked me more when I handled things. But it limited me. I put out fires and I was stuck in that role. I was giving my creative power away and constantly selling myself short.

Can you see how maybe a strength or something you pride yourself in may also show up as a weakness? We will come back to this topic in Chapter 7.

I have, it seems, always been attuned to the different voices in my head. "The witness" is something we speak of a lot in yoga. There is you, and then there is the part of you who sees you. It's very easy to disregard the inner voices or guides. Once I realized pretty much everything had to change in order for me to get well, the first thing I had to do was to stop doing. In fact, I didn't just have to stop doing, I had to start *Undoing* all the knots, to turn my attention to the things I had shoved away. It was consuming huge amounts of energy keeping myself in line.

I knew I was in total survivor mode. Just getting through each day was exhausting. Here is the thing about survival mode: every action is just a reaction to your environment, and usually we make bad decisions when we are just reacting. I knew all this – I had been teaching it for years, and yet here I was, finding out what it really meant to waive the white flag of surrender. I basically had to stop putting everyone else's needs above mine.

My first step needed to be subtle and soft. I simply made a commitment to myself to start taking a bath in essential oil-infused, nutrient-dense salts and seaweeds. Every time I got in the bath, it was as though I had pressed a little pause button.

I loved my baths. It was a way for me to retreat for a few minutes. I would feel instant relief in the Big Pause, and I realized I needed to spend some time noticing this tendency to keep pushing, no matter. Before I could make any specific changes, I wanted to notice just how much it was showing up in my life. I knew my choice: either I could continue with a familiar pattern that wasn't working for me, or I could rely on my knowledge from 20 years working and teaching in the spa and wellness industry to build a new pattern, a new way of being. I had to treat myself as I would a client and student. I had to make my health top priority, not because I wanted to be selfish, but because I wanted to fulfill my purpose in the world. I wanted to be available to serve and love my family, my students, and my community, which I couldn't possibly do until I restored my energy and health.

It doesn't matter what excuses you may have or I had. At the end of the day this vessel – body, mind, and heart – couldn't possibly support me the way I wanted it to if I didn't support it.

In owning my *dharma*, or purpose, I had to access my power, and the only way I could do that was to tend to what was quite obviously affecting every aspect of my life: my health.

Obviously you are reading this book because you are looking for answers, and you know you cannot continue the way that you have been going. Journaling is a very effective strategy for becoming clearer with your inner realm. Just because you write something down does not mean it is true, but it gives you the opportunity to really become aware of some of the background noise. In addition to that, it gives you a chance to practice communicating from the heart without fear. Take a moment to get a journal or notebook. I'm going to ask you some questions.

Before we start, pause for a few breaths and feel your body. Notice the quality of your mind: Is it busy, quiet, etc.? Move on to feeling your heart, your emotions.

Now, write down the answers to the following questions:

- Why do you think right now is the time to address your health?
- How is the way you feel every day stopping you from living the way you want? How does it show up with your kids, in your relationships, in your career?
- What is the inner dialogue you have when you feel like you might disappoint someone?

Remember, there is no right answer. It is just a time for reflection.

Now again, close your eyes, and feel a sense of gratitude for already having stepped towards wellness.

As you read through the following chapters, start to listen to the wisdom of your body. Trust it, and pay attention when it calls to you. Try to move into a space of wonder with your symptoms: Can you hear the message or feel the potential that change may bring? Think about stories of the great and inspiring people of history. They usually had some times of great adversity that grew them into the wise, inspirational people they became. This is your adversity. This is your time to grow.

After realizing I couldn't muscle my way through Hashimoto's, I knew there had to be another way. I used the following steps, and I know they will help you, too. These are my 6 steps to building the energy you need to create a life of wellness and joy.

The Big Pause

Pausing gives you the ability to become clear on your actions, what thoughts are behind the actions, and the choices you usually make. It is vitally important to give yourself the time to pause and reflect before adding more information.

Rest or Relax

Choosing rest is a vital part of the healing process. We have to switch off our stress response and move into a place of relaxation so the body can heal. You may be surprised to realize most of the things you do to relax are not rest, and that there is a difference.

Courage

Putting yourself first takes a great amount of courage. It is important to build your relationship with what your heart desires and to stop doing it without clear direction. Sometimes it takes the most courage to just feel what there is to be felt, with the only action to hold space for it.

Love and the Heart

Reconnect with your heart. Learn ways to support the emotional body, and practice what will help move things that you may have been holding for a while.

Inner Knowing

For most of your life thus far, you may have been pushing this little voice inside of you away, but now you will learn how to turn to it. Maybe for the first time in your life, learn how to show up for yourself, not because you should, but because you trust yourself.

Evolve

The un-doing process to reclaiming your energy takes action, but the actions are incredibly simple on purpose. The fastest way to lose all your energy all over again and end up back at the starting gate is to get ahead of yourself. Remember, this is about building the energy. Even as you start to notice things shift, you can just continue to let it build. You are so used to running on fumes, you will have a tendency to feel full even when your capacity is just beginning to grow. Hold steady and work the steps. If you are feeling great and taking on more, remain vigilant and pause frequently to check in. If you start to feel a little exhausted again, slow down. This is a process that will serve you for the rest of your life. You will begin to know what you need to do to collect and store more energy, and when you go through times in your life when you have to put out 110 percent for a while, you will know how to make sure you spend the extra time filling back up. An empty well = exhaustion, overwhelm, and reactivity.

I had a client, Jenn, who had so much going for her in so many ways, but she kept making it impossible for her to feel anything but exhaustion and overwhelm. The moment she created any space in her life, she filled it with something else. Pushing herself to the edge. She had done some work and come quite far, but I noticed she was starting to fall back. She had started telling herself the old way would be easier. She couldn't let go of the habit to just keep pushing, and this habit had now infiltrated every aspect of her life. She had the tools, but instead of using them as a key to the door, she was just running at the door. No amount of force would open it: she needed to soften and use the key. But it takes practice. We become so used to it being hard, to our old patterns and to being in overwhelm, that to soften feels foreign and scary. We actually begin to feel again as opposed to being in survival mode, shut down and reactionary. Jenn had to recommit to creating some space in her life. She realized that as she continued to push, things just got worse. It became so apparent that there was no other way but to start trusting and soften. What she had been doing was not working for her, and yet there was an attachment to it. It was scary for her to move away from her perceived strength, and yet she knew it was much scarier to stay where she was.

Just think for a moment how frustrating traffic can be when you are late. It seems like you catch every red light and encounter every bad driver in town. Contrast that with when you know you will be early to an appointment. You have space, traffic flows smoothly, you are compassionate to the people you notice struggling around you, and you actually notice the beauty around you. This is the perfect analogy for you. Right now, you feel like you are late, and everybody is doing their best to get in your way. We have to inject space into your life, before anything else.

In the case of autoimmune disease, our tendency is to try and understand what's wrong and how we can fix it. While this is an incredibly important piece of the puzzle, in this book you will learn to tap into your innate wisdom. To build the relationship between the many layers of your being and the most effective tools to create and live the life you desire.

We keep looking for the magic solution. Thinking that the next doctor or the next pill will work better. What would you say if I invited you to shift the direction, to look to your body for guidance first? Learn how to take stock of your energy, to understand the things that will increase your energy and the things that will take you down. The more you understand you, the greater your ability to engage with what you are feeling and the easier it will be to implement changes that feel life-affirming instead of restrictive and difficult.

Autoimmune disease can be literally about just surviving, but this is not somewhere you want to stay. It is possible to get to the other side of this equation. While your autoimmune disease may or may not go away, you are actually in a place of power. You can work and engage with it instead of just succumbing to whatever you feel every day and falling victim to it. I know it sucks! I have been there, and it is hard, but the sooner you begin to courageously understand that you have choices and consciously choose yourself, the sooner you will move beyond your wildest dreams. This is a catalyst for change if you choose it.

Chapter 2

The Big Pause

"So many of us are leading limited lives not because we have to but because we think we have to."

BRUCE LIPTON

Hashimoto's and too much stress tend to go hand-in-hand. If you're like me, on the days you have high energy you pack those hours full of things to do. How hard can I push today to get through my list in case tomorrow may not be so good? The first step in handling Hashimoto's is to Pause. Yes you heard that right, slow down and stop doing so much. Just for a little while!

I know you are probably wondering how you are going to fix this by not doing anything. Well, actually you are doing something: you are Pausing. Learning to slow down a little bit will help you develop a steadiness. When we have been under pressure, stress, and developing health issues for a while, we are usually operating from reactivity and fear, but the only way to see this clearly is to slow down. Imagine driving through a national park. You wouldn't drive as fast as possible to get through, you would drive slowly, pausing periodically to take a picture or just to take in your surroundings. This is the feeling I want you to try to create as you build Pause into your life. A sense of just starting to notice all that is beneath the surface.

One of the most important steps and something I encourage you not to rush through is this one. Stop. I know that may feel a bit counter-intuitive. Imagine for a moment that you are driving to a friend's house, one you haven't been to before. You think you have followed the directions perfectly, and yet you have not arrived at the correct house. You assume you must have done something wrong, so you go back to your house and start again, following the exact same directions. Again, you end up at the wrong house.

How many times would you do this before realizing that you were not the problem, and so it must be the directions? To remedy the situation, the first thing you would need to do is stop the pattern – in this case, following incorrect directions. Then, and only then, could you decide what to do next, whether you wait until you can get your friend on the phone, or just go home. You see now that it doesn't matter that you thought you had the right directions or that you did everything right. When you stop, you give yourself the opportunity to approach the problem differently. In the case of Hashimoto's, it allows you to notice what you are feeling. With every decision you make, it is a great practice to learn to first pause and notice where the answer is coming from. Try not to add negative self-talk to the Big Pause; it is not with judgment we ask the question, it is with curiosity and wonder. I wonder why I want that cookie so much....

Stress is stress, it doesn't make any difference to the body whether you are worrying about your finances, the decisions your child is making, or the physical stress you feel because you ache all over. Some days, it is all you can do to get through until bedtime. What's happening tomorrow, next week, or next month doesn't even register, because it can't. As you read the following chapters, you will be reminded of what it really means to rest and how difficult that is if you don't make it a priority.

It is the human condition to have a to-do list too big to complete. As we finish one thing, we see another pop up. Is all this busy-ness getting you where you want to go? I'm going to assume the answer is no, or you wouldn't be reading this book. It seems that busy-ness has become normal, everyday life for us as women. There is no denying we have a lot to do. From the house, to taking care of the kids, to our careers, and now maintaining our health. Let's face it: Something usually has to give, and that thing is usually us.

Burnt Toast Syndrome

We suffer from burnt toast syndrome. You know, when you eat the burnt toast or the food that fell on the floor and give your children or husband all the best stuff. I totally had burnt toast syndrome! The syndrome goes so much deeper into our lives and the relationships we have with our loved ones. It's vitally important for you to never eat burnt toast again! You see, when we don't value ourselves, we are putting a message out to everyone else that we don't matter as much. We are sending a message to the universe and reinforcing the inner dialogue that everyone else is more important than us.

I am a big believer that the way we treat ourselves sets the tone for how we will be received and treated. No wonder it is so difficult for us to take the time to nurture ourselves! For so long, we have been giving ourselves the message that what we are feeling or desiring is not important as long as everyone else is happy. When we Pause, it gives us the opportunity to remember our sustenance is important; the food we eat gives us the ability to continue to show up for ourselves and the people we love most. I can remember not only eating burnt toast, but also the sandwich crusts I cut off for my kids and the leftover scraps on their plate most of the time because of my busy-ness. In trying to make it easy on myself, I actually made it harder. Trying to function optimally without proper nourishment is very difficult to do.

As mothers, we tend to pride ourselves on being able to do it all. Most of the time, we will push and push until the point of exhaustion, and then we will keep pushing because we don't know what else to do. Once burn-out sets in, it's difficult to recover. It is quite a phenomenon really. For the most part, we are the oil that keeps the machine moving, yet we don't find it important to put ourselves first. I am not that great at getting my car tuned up at 30,000, 60,000 or even 100,000 miles, but I do get my oil changed when it is needed for two reasons: 1) I know it's a relatively small investment of time and not much hassle, and 2) I know one sure way to blow an engine quickly is to run out of oil.

We are constantly pushing ourselves to do more and we need to take the time to re-nourish ourselves. Pause allows us time to disengage with our habitual patterns, and by doing that, we are then able to reset the system. Any action taken before pausing will probably be more of the same.

Your Pitcher

Imagine yourself as a pitcher of water. The water that fills you equates to your energy. Every action, thought, and breath takes energy. In a perfect world, every night as you sleep the body gets detoxed, and the pitcher gets refilled. You wake up in the morning, and your pitcher is full because you slept well and you have been taking good care of yourself. You are ready for a new day.

But if you stayed up too late working or trying to catch up on a few last to-dos or you binge-watched TV, you may find yourself waking up to a half-full pitcher. Now, can you imagine the difference you will feel if you start your day with a half-full pitcher versus a full one? What happens when you run out of water, but you are only halfway through your day? Well, that depends on you, but Pausing gives you the opportunity to name what you are feeling. Instead of craving chocolate and coffee, you realize you are tired and your water, or energy, is depleted.

This Pause is key to helping us shift what we do next. When we learn to see the thought behind the action, we are no longer victim to weak willpower. We learn to find a way to refill our container with a short rest or some energy-building food instead of a quick source of energy like sugar or caffeine, which will just give us a short burst but will cost more energy later to detox. This in essence puts us into borrowed water. Our bodies will respond to the call to action by moving us into a state of stress. Basically you are borrowing from your emergency fund.

Now, our wise bodies have some crisis management systems in place. The problem occurs when we get used to crisis management and start to live in it. Putting your body into a state of stress makes your adrenal glands work harder to produce the hormones that will keep you moving. This is why so many people experience lack of willpower, adrenal fatigue, or burn-out. Can you see how this process will continue to run us in the red? It is not sustainable, and the body's stress response is not meant to be in constant engagement.

Oftentimes, what drains our pitcher is the amount of things we worry about. *How am I going to pay the bills?* or *How am I going to get this all done?* are two common examples of thoughts that can actually deplete our water faster. We worry, and we forget that there is something so much more valuable than money or accomplishment: our health. For when we are healthy and have lots of energy, we feel big and capable. We are inspired and enthusiastic about life; we are a force to be reckoned with. Additional rest and better sleep schedules build our capacity to hold more water, and we will continue to grow the size of our pitcher, making it possible for us to have days of stress and high activity without running into the negative.

This is where the Big Pause comes in. I call it the Big Pause because I know when I ask you to stop, at first you cannot understand how this will help. I get it. You have a lot on your plate. But remember, by doing this you are on your way to building yourself a bigger container. In fact, as you can see from the water pitcher example, it is very difficult to do anything in your life at your highest potential if you are limited by the size of your reservoir.

It seems a rather simple action to pause, but honestly, when we are acting from a place of reactivity, we usually make bad choices before we even realize what we are doing, and then chastise ourselves about it later. In this first step, we simply Pause to recognize the habitual behavior and to try and hear the thought that is attached to it. Don't be hard on yourself right now. The goal is not to start imposing actions on yourself to change behavior, but to notice the behavior and the feelings or thoughts attached to it.

About a year after my Hashimoto's diagnosis, I took a sabbatical. That sounds like I consciously decided, but you know it really wasn't that simple. I had owned a yoga studio for the previous five years and had been teaching and seeing clients privately six days a week – not to mention that I had to switch gears into mom-chauffeur mode pick up from school, transform into chef and cook dinner, become a teacher to help with homework, then morph back into mom for bedtime. From the moment I crawled out of bed in the morning to the moment I crawled back in, I was pushing through. I really believed that if I just kept pushing, things would eventually get easier, something would give.

But it didn't happen that way. The yoga studio's landlord was not willing to sign a lease, so we were on a month-to-month basis for some time. We had looked for other spaces, but strangely, it seemed they all got rented to someone else within moments of us putting in an offer. All the signs were there that this would be the perfect opportunity to close the business, slow down a little bit, and take some time to rebuild my health. But I just couldn't seem to let go.

My sister, who was also my business partner, was ready to close the business because it felt right for her. I still struggled. In fact, I was ready to take it on alone even though I was struggling with my health and already had too much on my plate. Why did I continue to push? What was it that made me unaware of the space this would give me? Or was it the very space that felt so scary?

My sister and I were scheduled to travel to Colorado to study with our teacher, and it was just the break I needed to get some perspective. I had the opportunity to talk with my teacher about what I was feeling; this time away gave me the opportunity to be in contemplation. This, in essence, was a Big Pause for me. It gave me the space to ask the question: *why?* Why did I need to push through? I didn't come home with total resolve; it took time to be willing to put things down for a while. But I knew I needed to put myself first.

I didn't tell you that story because I want you to make a radical change in your life right now, but because I want you to give yourself the space to see where you might need it. To notice if there is something you are pushing away with fervor, or if you are pushing through like a bulldozer. I know firsthand that once you start to have issues with your health, you can only pretend everything is ok for a little while and then the need to fix it becomes strong. Statistically speaking, once you have one autoimmune condition, the chances of getting another one escalates significantly. Try not to let that scare you. Instead, use it to motivate yourself to hear the call to change. The most important thing right now is to add the Big Pause and listen to what the space has to tell you.

My client Beth used to crash every day at about 3 o'clock. She would pick her kids up from school, go home and get them a snack, and then collapse in her room to watch TV for a while until she had to make dinner or couldn't put off work another moment. Together we were able to recognize the wall she hit every afternoon. Beth began to insert a Pause here. Just a few moments of recognizing the exhaustion gave her the ability to see it for what it was. In the past, she had just wanted to check out – watch TV, eat a little sugar, and drink some caffeine until she had enough perceived energy to push through the rest of the day. The Big Pause helped Beth to notice her exhaustion. Instead of pushing it away, she could soften to it. Beth now knew it would happen and could start to build strategies that would help her.

Pretending to be anything that you are not takes energy, and so you see the moment you allow yourself to just feel and notice where you are, space is created. Within this space, comes the potential for change.

Pause = Space

Space = Potential

Let me clarify that for a moment. If you continue to operate from a place of stress, you will continue to make decisions from the reactive brain, which wants immediate gratification. Inserting a Pause will not help you to change that yet, but it will begin to let you see your habitual patterns and how you are repeatedly sabotaging your dreams. It's actually an improvement to move into a conscious "bad" choice and out of the subconscious. It also gives you the ability, as we move further into the book, to interrupt the pattern entirely and make better choices.

I remember when I was first playing with this idea myself. I was in the bakery section at Whole Foods, and they had some really lovely cookies. I wanted one, but because I was able to Pause, I noticed that my desire for the cookie was because I was actually feeling depleted, and it shifted that craving for chocolate to a desire for more energy. I still ate the cookie, and it gave me a quick boost – but I also noticed the crash later. This helped me start to see the pattern of high and low energy I had through the day. A desire for energy came up as a sugar craving. I had them all the time. But with this new information I got from pausing, I was able to actually rename the desire. No longer was it about sugar, but about energy and while I knew sugar would be a quick source of energy, right around the corner would be a crash and another craving.

Again, don't jump to the change part. First, we must create the space. From this space comes the ability to create and change. It is, however, our tendency, as we talked about earlier, to be busy and the moment we create a little space we tend to fill it with something, anything. Remember my client Jenn, who was creating more space but kept filling it with more and more to do's? She didn't know how to exist in space and was habitually running on stress. Space can in some ways be uncomfortable. We look for things to distract us and put pressure on ourselves because we think it keeps us in our comfort zone, but our bodies are telling a different story. This frenetic pace is not so comfortable! This is the crazy thing: When we fill the space unconsciously, it will usually be with something that is not going to help us. Again, it is using the reactive brain and not the cognitive brain. So as you incorporate space into your thoughts and into your life, consider it precious stuff and store it up like a squirrel preparing for winter.

Setting Your Intention and Creating Space for Change

One of the best ways I have found to set the intention for creating space is to start and finish every day with a Pause. You may think this sounds easy, but believe me, it is incredibly easy to forget. I recommend when you first implement this step you link it to something else you do habitually every day, like brushing your teeth. If you're like most of us, you brush your teeth at least twice a day and sometimes more than that, so at first it's a good idea to attach the Big Pause to brushing your teeth.

I would also link your Pause to an essential oil blend (this is not necessary but it is helpful) something calming like frankincense or lavender. Every morning when you go to the sink to brush your teeth, pick up your oil instead. Place two drops in the palms of your hands and take a few deep breaths. Then say a little prayer, something like, "May I be present to all that I feel today, and may I remember to pause and listen to my heart." Make it your own, and remember that it's really not what you say, but what the intention is behind what you say. Every time you brush your teeth, remember to do this ritual first.

Expanding the Big Pause with Breath

As you get more and more comfortable with your intention-setting, you can begin to build it into a short breath practice. A breath practice is a fantastic way to have direct access to your nervous system. When you first start working with breath, it is best to keep it nice and simple. I love the one-to-one breath, and it goes like this:

Close your eyes and count the length of your inhale, but don't go to your fullest ability. I recommend a four-second inhale to start. As you exhale, make the length of your exhale be the same length as your inhale. As you continue to breathe, just continue to count the breath. Inhale 2 3 4. Exhale 2 3 4. See if you can relax even more and make your breath smoother. If your mind starts to wander, just pull it back to the breath. Get interested and curious, don't try to force anything. This breath will help you build more steadiness and ease, which is absolutely foundational to lasting change. As we work to build stability, you will move more and more away from the ups and downs of stress naturally.

This practice only works if you do it daily but keep it short at first so you won't tell yourself it's something you're too busy to do. Commit to intentional breathing for three to five minutes every morning before you get dressed. Set your alarm five minutes earlier so you can do this practice. Ideally sit in the same seat at the same time. As you finish your practice, say thank you to yourself for making and keeping the commitment.

Chapter 3

Rest

*"Allow yourself to rest. Your soul speaks to you in
the quiet moments in between your thoughts."*

UNKNOWN

Once you begin to insert the Big Pause into your daily life, you will become more aware of the underlying experience of what is propelling you through each day. I recommend just taking note in that pause. Notice how you are feeling.

Imagine for a moment that your child comes to you and says, "Mommy, I'm really tired." What kind of advice would you give? Would you tell them to have a donut and a coffee, and that they would have more energy soon? Would you say, "Oh, honey, I'm so sorry, would you like a treat?" Or would you say something more like, "Ok, baby, let's get you some decent food and you can lie down for a little while."?

It's an important step to begin to name exactly what you are feeling so that you can create an action response that is appropriate. Use this method of speaking to your child as a technique to teach yourself to be gentle with yourself. We feel compassion and love towards our children when they come to us with feelings. Treat yourself with that same compassion. Begin to hear the difference between the old self-talk and how you shift your self-talk using this technique. It's amazing how hard we can be on ourselves.

If you notice you are exhausted or tired, then the appropriate action is to schedule rest times in your day. Remember my client Beth, who noticed every afternoon she would hit a wall at 3:00 pm? If you know these walls are up ahead, then why not take action to prevent hitting them? I recommend at the very least scheduling a few minutes to relax, close your eyes, and take some deep breaths – better yet, take 15-20 minutes to do a relaxing Yoga Nidra. (Check out my recorded one at leahcarver. com.)

I have found that, left to our own devices, most of us don't know how to rest. Instead of getting actual sleep, for example, we think watching TV or having a glass of wine will help us – and while they might help us relax and can stop the mind, they are not building energy. Here is the thing: our bodies are designed in such a way that we are constantly in communication from our inner environment to our outer environment, filtering and processing information. This complex system is called our nervous system. Our senses – sight, sound, smell, taste, and touch – are always picking up information and sending messages to the brain. The activities we consider relaxing can actually be quite stressful on the body and brain.

Take TV, for example. There are sounds and lights we are filtering, a story line we are following, and then we are having an emotional response to the story lines, meaning we are literally living them. If it's funny, we are laughing right along with the TV; if it's sad, we may be crying. This is actually one reason we watch TV: to create an opportunity to leave what we are feeling and go somewhere else or maybe we just want a good excuse to cry. I am not against watching a good movie. But remember, while it may be relaxing, it is not rest.

I can remember back a few years ago by the time I would get my kids to bed and the house organized enough for the next morning, I would be exhausted and climb into bed. I wouldn't go to sleep, though. Instead, I would start watching something on TV. It felt like the ultimate indulgence – everyone was asleep and I could just check out. Of course this often meant I would stay up too late and be dragging and slightly moody when I got up in the morning. I find now I no longer want to watch TV very often. It wasn't that I had to discipline myself to stop watching, it was literally as soon as I felt better and my energy was up, I no longer found it interesting.

It seems the other go-to is drinking alcohol. I get it, it can help us relax. While this is ok, it would be a good idea to cut alcohol out for the next six weeks while you work through Undoing. It will give you the opportunity to see how you feel without it. It seems society pairs alcohol with almost everything: cooking dinner, watching a game, hanging out at the beach, going out with friends, parties, fundraisers, brunch

– the list just keeps on going. Why? Because it gets us to relax. We lighten up and let go of our inhibitions. Drinking keeps our minds distracted so we don't have to feel what we are feeling.

The problem is, the escape doesn't last. Often, we feel anxiety after drinking, and our bodies have to process the toxins and consume much of our energy to do so. Instead, see if you can take some deep breaths and lighten up, try to feel a sense of ease about it all. I want to be clear here and reinforce that I am not saying you shouldn't drink a glass of wine occasionally. What I am recommending is that you start to get interested in what feelings come with the desire to have a glass of wine. Ask yourself what it is you like about wine: how does it help you relax, what are the qualities of the relaxation you get from it? If you stop having wine to relax, then it may help you to develop other techniques to unwind. But if you always drink wine in the evening to relax, you will probably have a more difficult time relaxing without it. It's just like a baby and a pacifier. You know they can sleep without it, but they don't know that. You have to teach them.

The quote at the beginning of the chapter gives us guidance into understanding that when we are feeling rested, we start to connect with our deeper sense of self. We can hear our desires and dreams, and access a place of creativity.

Rest is having the opportunity to just be. To notice, to feel, and to stop doing. I used to tell my kids, "Mommy needs a little time to rest," leaving my eldest in charge. I'd go into my room, climb into bed, and watch TV. I would get up a little later, but I would not feel rested. I wanted to stay in my bed and not move.

This all changed when I applied better strategies for resting and actually allowing my body some recovery time.

Here are some very helpful strategies for resting: turn off sensory stimulation, connect to yourself or nature, or try taking some deep breaths. We often limit ourselves with the idea that we don't have time to rest, but if we learn to manage rest sessions in a way that rebuilds our energy, we will find ourselves much more capable of not just performing our duties for the rest of the day, but actually feeling more vibrant and available.

Within the Autonomic Nervous System, there are two branches: the sympathetic nervous system (SNS) and the parasympathetic nervous system (PSNS). The SNS is the area of the "fight or flight" response, the part of our nervous system that functions while we are under stress. Adrenaline is increased, we have more speed, strength, and physical ability so that we can fight for survival or run like mad. This is why people have been able to do super-human things in extremely stressful situations, like lifting a car off someone. In addition to adrenaline, norepinephrine is produced, which increases alertness. Have you ever been driving late at night, feeling a little tired, and hit a pothole or a dip in the road? All of a sudden, you are much more awake. Finally, the Sympathetic Nervous System produces cortisol. Cortisol is one of the most talked-about adrenal hormones. It can be life-saving in acute stress as it works to regulate blood pressure and other important bodily functions. In chronic stress, however, the body just continues to release cortisol, and this can lead to bigger problems.

The ParaSympathetic Nervous System, on the other hand, is the "rest and digest" side. This governs our ability to relax and recover. When we are in a sympathetic (SNS) state, we are not able to rest, digest, or heal as well. Think about how common stress-related stomach issues are, from a so-called "nervous stomach" to an ulcer or Irritable Bowel Syndrome (IBS). Statistics say 80 percent of disease is caused by stress. My mother and well known spa educator Anne Bramham always said that "the doctors can have the 20 percent and the spas can take care of the stress."

A great tool to help you increase your capacity for change and greater self discipline is to learn how to shift out of sympathetic into a parasympathetic state. As I mentioned earlier, when you insert the Big Pause, you will build awareness of where the thoughts that dictate your behavior are coming from. If you have been operating in the sympathetic state, meaning from stress, exhaustion, and overwhelm, for a while (like most of your life?), you may need to teach your body how to switch into a parasympathetic state. A great example of this is parenting. As mothers, we teach babies how to relax and fall asleep by giving them a bedtime routine: a relaxing massage, gentle music, rocking, and holding them close to feel our heart beat. All of these things help them begin to relax.

Another key component here is digestion. Often we eat without taking the time to stop what we are doing and be present. We are not giving our bodies the ability to properly digest and absorb the food we are consuming when we eat on the go or with little awareness. Eating low-quality and low-vibrancy food tends to go hand-in-hand with not paying attention.

Remember why we eat. First and foremost, we eat to give our bodies sustainable energy. If we can begin to change the way we engage with mealtime and see it with a sense of reverence and as an opportunity to increase our power, we will find the results to be incredible. Make eating not just an afterthought, but actually one of the most important things you do every day. Picture this: you are at work and your morning appointment ran over. You have about 20 minutes before your next one and you are starving. What will you grab to eat? Even as I ask this question, having not had grains or sugar in ages, my mind still jumps immediately to Starbucks. Grab a coffee and a pastry to tide me over, keep me going. It is quite obvious if you visit Starbucks in the morning that there are a lot of people who think like me. So while you have filled your stomach, you have actually gone into an energy deficit. Sugar and caffeine will keep you going, but I guarantee you will have a crash. Jump forward in your day, how do you get though the next crash? Can you see how this pattern precipitates exhaustion? So instead of setting yourself up for failure, make a plan, just like you schedule your appointments at work. Set a clear boundary, make your lunch time valuable, and don't let the meeting go over. Bring something you can eat that will take less time, or have a local healthy restaurant on speed dial. Even if it's a little more expensive, it will be worth it.

The thoughts you connect to the choices you make are also incredibly important. Do you come from a place of negative or positive self-talk? You can change "I shouldn't eat that," or "If I eat that I will be a bad girl," etc. to something more like, "If I make good choices now, I will build my energy, feel empowered, and be available for fun and connection with my family later."

Our bodies are in constant communication with both our external environment and internal environment. They are a physical manifestation of what is going on internally, and what's going on externally will also create internal changes. They are a vitally important part of being able to live our purpose. If you come to life from a place of depletion and are living from a state of stress, you will be limited in what you can achieve, as opposed to if you were vibrant, healthy, and well. Revere your body and it will serve you.

Think of your body as the place that receives and delivers messages. We get very clear signals of what is going on and when something is wrong. But when we have lived under high stress for too long, we no longer hear the signals, and they just become background noise we have learned to tune out.

Sometimes the simple answer is not what we choose. We think it has to be hard. We may say, "Rest? Who has time for rest?" and then schedule a surgery that requires radical lifestyle changes, when in actuality if we give our body the break it needs, then we are at least giving it an opportunity to heal. The parasympathetic or rest state is when the body heals itself. Everything in the body is connected like a woven web or matrix. If there is an issue in one part of your body, it will affect the rest; the body is a whole. Removing one malfunctioning organ via surgery may not fix the whole problem.

A friend of mine who is an incredible health coach told me about a client of his who had come to him with severe digestive issues. While going through her medical history, she told him she had her large intestine removed. His recommendation at the end of the session was to eat mostly a liquid diet – juiced vegetables, soups, etc. She said to him, "Don't you think that's a bit drastic?"

His reply was, "I told you to eat vegetables and you think that's drastic, but you let a surgeon remove your large intestine without even a second opinion?" Sometimes we tend to act before we even see all of the options, and a lot of the time what appears to be the quick fix actually comes with its own limitations. I'm not advocating for not having medical procedures but I am recommending you ask what happens next and get a few opinions.

While medication may be necessary, it should not be treated as a complete fix. Going on a medication for the rest of your life should not be something we jump to. First, I believe it is important to ask why there is a problem and learn the lifestyle changes that will support healing it. In the case of Hashi's, medication does not fix the autoimmune problem, it only supports the body by providing the hormones your thyroid is not producing.

One of the problems we usually face is that by the time we feel enough pain to get our attention, it is usually going to take a little bit more effort to recover. Chances are, this has been going on for some time, and so it will take time to heal. I am in no way saying not to take medication; what I am saying is don't stop there. Keep working the problem, get to the bottom of it, and make the lifestyle changes that will support you on a happy, healthy journey.

Rest is a big part of the equation. The body only heals itself in a deep place of relaxation or sleep. Think about your child. When they get sick, it is their instinctive reaction to go to bed and sleep. They sleep a lot. A few days later, they are up and running. As adults, we think we can't possibly sleep for a few days, even when we know that is exactly what we need. We have jobs to do, children to take care of, etc. We don't give ourselves the opportunity to get well. It usually has to be something big to get that kind of attention, but if we ignore the problems long enough, that is exactly what we end up with. Getting a good night sleep is vital to our health. It really gives us the opportunity to detox and restore our energy from the day before. Can you see the problem here? Nobody really takes the time to rest, and even when we do, we don't know how to do it effectively.

My client Stephanie was going through an incredibly stressful time in her life and her Hashimoto's, which hadn't been bothering her, was acting up. She was feeling old and creaky in her joints, though she was only in her early 40s, and she had developed a chronic dry cough. As things neared a complete breaking point, the weekend getaway she had planned months ago was right around the corner. Her thought was to cancel the trip, as she was worried being away would make the stress worse. But she was able to Pause and realize she needed to rest. She went off on her trip, and there happened to be a spa close by that had a sauna and cold plunge. She decided to spend the first afternoon there. She followed a protocol I recommended. As she left the spa, she felt great, but soon after arriving back at her hotel, she started to feel flu-like symptoms. Both cold and feverish, she was exhausted and crashed in bed for two hours. When she woke up, she felt amazing. Stephanie spent the next three days in complete rest and relaxation. She found that when she arrived home, she was much better able to deal with the stress, and while things were not perfect, the fact that she had spent three days building up her reservoir again meant she had much more focus and was able to make better choices.

The really great news is that while nothing quite compares to the spa experience of contrasting hot and cold treatments, we can support these actions on a daily basis in our homes. It is simple, effective lifestyle support.

Bathing

The history books tell of the Roman Empire's invasion of Europe. As they settled along the war path, they stayed only in areas of running water and natural springs. The sanitation standards of the Roman Empire were not the same after its demise, and remained in that sorry state until after WWII. Much of Roman society and culture was based around the ritual of bathing. There is a lot to know about why water can be such a powerful tool when used for better health. First of all, think of the natural desire to shower to wash the day off, or the desire to go on vacation to the beach, a lake, or hiking near a waterfall. We have a natural yearning toward water, a wise and innate instinct.

Water is one of the best conductors of energy. Think about how often you use water to conduct heat and cook. When we immerse ourselves in water, we surround our internal water environment with an external water environment. This allows us to use temperature to manipulate a specific body response. Heat increases circulation, or the movement of blood, which in turn increases the rate at which oxygen and nutrients are delivered throughout the body. A short application of cold will encourage the blood to rush away from the surface to the deeper organs, which also means a carrying away of waste from an area. The body in its creation is rather spectacular, and it is my opinion if we just give it the opportunity to do what it does best by cleaning up the inner environment and giving it the nutrients and biochemical elements it needs to be healthy, then it will work to get us back on the path to wellness.

Another attribute of water is to act as a solvent, meaning its ability to dissolve and distribute products like salt or seaweed powders in it. This means that as we soak in our tub we can determine what minerals we want/need to support the issues or symptoms we are managing. One of the functions of the skin is absorption. This is exciting because it means that while we are struggling with our health and our doctors have probably recommended we start taking a slew of supplements, we can, in additional to running tests on our gut health, look to the bath to help support our intake of minerals and bio-chemical elements. Not to mention the fact that taking a bath should feel a little like a retreat, some time to just rest and re-nourish.

Hydrotherapy, or water therapy, is an amazing tool traced back to ancient Rome. It gets our blood moving. When we do hot and cold therapies, we induce a parasympathetic state. It gives us a way of meeting the body where it is in intensity and dropping us into quiet and calm, moving us from sympathetic to a parasympathetic state. One of my favorite practices for relaxing the nervous system is to take a neutral temperature bath about 97 degrees with Epsom salt or other natural and nourishing ingredients. It won't feel cold, but it won't heat the body up and cause sedation. The body sees the neutral temperature as very stabilizing.

You have begun the journey of listening to the body, collecting information, and responding to this internal information-gathering. We then have to put into practice ways of addressing what we are noticing. The key is to first identify that there is a problem, and what you are doing now is not helping. Then simply try a few different strategies to find something that will help you rest your body and mind. You will begin to rest, and may fall asleep – or at the very least get a deep sense of rest. Remember one of the best things you can do to help yourself feel better and have more energy is to give your body the opportunity to digest all the information it receives, including food, from the day. While we rest, the body detoxifies itself. If we don't get enough rest, the body is more likely to store toxins and other information not fully digested. The greater toxic load you have to burn up, the more rest you will require as your body will be working harder.

Breath and the Nervous System

You may have caught the line in the previous chapter where I said the breath is a direct link to the nervous system. I want to take just a little more time to discuss this with you. In your life, you may see this every day. Do you notice how irregular your breath may get when you are feeling frustrated or upset? People who suffer with anxiety or panic attacks often experience a sense of hyperventilating. When someone experiences a shock, we usually coach them to calm down and take some deep breaths. It's because when we can start to regulate the breath, we send a message to the heart and then the nervous system that all is ok. We encourage our bodies to switch out of sympathetic mode and into parasympathetic mode. As you practiced the circular breath, you probably noticed that either the inhale or the exhale was easier. When we want to create a relaxation response, it's best to use a longer exhale.

So close your eyes right now, and start with balanced breath. Now, every time you exhale, lengthen your exhale for one count. So if you inhale for a count three, exhale for a count of four. Then inhale for three and exhale for five. Inhale for three, and exhale for six. Continue with this breathing pattern, inhaling for one count, exhaling for two.

Another practice that is incredibly calming is a heating compress. Dip a washcloth in ice cold water, wring it out, and apply it to your belly. Cover it with a dry towel, and then cover up with a blanket – preferably wool or some other fiber that will retain heat. Lie down and rest for 20 minutes.

Chapter 4

Build

*"Let today be the day you love yourself enough
to no longer just dream of a better life; let it be
the day you act upon it."*

STEVE MARABOLI

Recently, I was working with a client and when I asked what it was she really wanted or what goal she had in mind for the next year, she wasn't able to clearly come up with anything except that she wanted to feel better, but was already worried about the effort that would take.

It takes a lot of courage to remind yourself of what you desire. It means at times choosing what appears to be the more difficult road, although you may find this road holds many secret inspirations. It's choosing the path of your soul, and to choose it consistently takes being brave.

As you reflect on the difficulty of keeping commitments to yourself in regard to your health and wellness, you may notice some fear there. What if you just can't make the lifestyle changes you need to make, what if you try and you don't feel any better? It takes courage to be gentle with yourself. We have unrealistic expectations of ourselves, and we feel guilt and shame when we can't take the actions we need to take. Give yourself some space and cultivate your ability to hold energy. See what it feels like to stop pushing so hard, and give yourself permission to have a recovery time of more than a few days.

For a moment, think about how fear may be playing a role in slowing down your process. Does it feel scary to you to make lifestyle changes? Do you worry about how your changes will inconvenience others or change the dynamic of your family and friend relationships?

This disease is pushing you out of your comfort zone. It is no longer comfortable to remain in old patterns, and yet it can feel very scary to change or step onto an unknown path. It takes some Pause and being brave to be able to see how we limit ourselves. We may hear that voice of judgment saying *I am not enough, I need to be able to eat the foods I know aren't good for me, I need to have a cocktail to relax and be fun, I probably won't be able to do it anyway.*

Get your journal, close your eyes for a few breaths, and then ask yourself the following questions:

- Why do I want to eat the foods I know don't make me feel well? (Spend a little time unpacking that and see if you can go underneath – is there another layer?)
- Why do I find it difficult to rest if that is what I need?
- What is one change I can make today that will help relieve some of my stress?
- What is my biggest fear with my Hashimoto's?

When you first start to build energy, it is like a small spark of fire. If you want the spark to turn into fire, you need a little tinder, and you need sticks and logs so it will transform into a long-sustaining fire. If the fire burns too hot too soon, you may not have the logs to support sustenance, and the fire will go out. It is very important that you get this: We must not take on too much just because we are reminded of our spark. Take some time to build up energy, store it and let it start to seep into every part of your being. With a small amount of energy, you will not be able to create a big fire, but if you wait and collect it, you will once again feel full and you will vibrate with life and energy.

Over and over again, I see with my clients that it's the old "two steps forward, one step back." They start to feel a bit better and all of a sudden are feeling creative, and then boom, they start to do too much. Before you know it, they have pushed too far and are left feeling energy-depleted once again.

Melissa was so scared of never reaching her goals. She always felt she was here to do something great, but by the time she came to work with me, she was so tired and couldn't think more than a few days ahead. I took her through my Undoing program, and after a few weeks she was feeling better, more like her old self. We had to spend a significant amount of time on this step, though, because Melissa was a Doer. The moment she started to feel better, she would quickly fill the space with something else. Jumping at each opportunity as it presented itself.

The problem Melissa was struggling with was that she still didn't have a good storehouse of energy. In one instance, she offered to throw a surprise party for a friend. She was excited about having everyone over and hosting the event. The party was a big success, but Melissa was exhausted. And it took her days to recover. It was a great lesson for her, though. She was able to see that even though she was feeling substantially better, her periods of high energy were still quite fleeting. She needed the courage to just stay in this place of feeling inspired without taking on any more, so she could feel her dreams reignite. Especially because Melissa was a Doer, it was very important she remain connected to the goal of energy-building. This was hard for her; she was excited and feeling fiery. It took courage to just hold steady and know that if she did too much too soon, she would burn herself out again.

My advice to Melissa was to slow down a little bit. To soften to the more subtle awareness of the energy she was now building. Get intimate with it, and notice where her highs and lows of energy were, and if there seemed to be fewer highs and lows and more consistent energy. Notice how falling asleep at night felt, and whether upon waking, she felt rejuvenated. It was important that she have a basic routine in place before she took on too much. A consistent bed time and a consistent time to wake and do her morning practice.

Once that's in place, this is when you can start to take action. In the meantime, reside in a place of power, tending to your needs and knowing you are on your way to your dreams. Spend time dreaming up what you want to create, and enjoy being in that space. What was truly exciting for Melissa is that as she got more capable of building energy, her goals and eventually her actions actually got bigger. She was able to step away from her family's business and start her own. She no longer needed to defer her power or have the safety net of other people.

Right now you may find yourself operating out of an energy deficit, and you are continually trying to find new ways to increase your energy so you can keep going. Hopefully, though, you are starting to understand the idea of energy as a commodity. It's time we look at balancing your energy much like you would your checkbook. In order to pay out money, you must have money in the account, or the check will not clear. As you take steps to build more energy, you can start putting some aside in a saving account. So now you have a checking and savings account. The saving account is there in case you need overdraft protection or for days when you know you won't be bringing in as much as you are putting out. The last and final part to understand is investing your energy in resources that will increase your return.

Here are some things I find inspire me and help me build energy: rest, spa diet, yoga and breath practice, baths, nature, hiking, the beach, communing with like-minded people, being inspired, and laughing and being silly. What do you like to do that makes you feel alive? Make a list of things you think will help build energy.

It is apparent when you feel well and have accounts full of energy. You perform at a level far beyond anything you can come close to when you are running on borrowed energy. Do you remember when I compared energy to the water pitcher earlier?

I want you to understand that I get it and we are all human. We will at times, especially if we are not careful, find ourselves energy-deficient once again. But once you learn these tools, most of the time that deficit will be from circumstances quite outside your control. Know that we are brilliantly designed, and our bodies can manage short stints of stress – but then we must restore. If you ignore this truth, you will soon find yourself once again in a place of extreme exhaustion and "pain," whether it be physical, mental, or emotional. Our society has created a situation where we feel busy, stressed, and overwhelmed too much of the time. We have never really been taught how to recover from everyday stress. Think about it: How has your life been for the last 5, 10, or maybe even 20 years? Have you had a running to-do list for as long as you can remember? Do you often feel like you just need it to stop?

Action without energy can look a lot like the definition of insanity – you know, doing the same thing over and over again and expecting different results. If you don't have the energy to back up what you are trying to do, then you will just waste what little energy you have on trying. Can you relate? Do you know someone who is constantly jumping from one project to another but never really accomplishing much? They have a great idea and feel totally inspired by it, but the next time you see them and ask about it, they say, "Oh, that, no, it just didn't work out." It is extremely common. Eventually these people may stop trying and just learn to deal with working a job that feels just ok. In the case of Hashimoto's, they may say, "Well, I tried that – changing my diet – but it was too much work and I felt deprived, so I stopped."

Do you see how we just keep setting ourselves up for failure? We will continue to do this until the point that we learn to do it differently – to see it coming and take actions to prevent it by building energy. Recognize the desire to make a big commitment – for example, changing the way you eat for the rest of your life. Then hold the desire close and think about it, how it feels to honor this commitment and how life will be different. Imagine yourself at parties: What will you eat? Start to think about all the things that will get in your way and see yourself able to keep the commitment in a way that feels easy. The desire to eat the food that makes you feel bad is fading, and your desire to eat healthy, vibrant food grows. There is no need to go on a "diet" – a diet sounds like something you do for a short while, but this is so much more powerful. This is lasting change. If you build your energy first, you will start to make better choices, and it doesn't feel restrictive. As you continue to build your energy, you will notice yourself making better choices more often in your life.

It is vital that you know what the goal is. For a moment reflect on one of the lifestyle changes you have tried to make in the past. Remember how you felt at the beginning of the commitment or resolution. Did you start with a feeling of dread, or was it just the next step? Chances are that if you didn't succeed, there may have been an underlying negative feeling or even pre-crafted excuses like "Well, if I can't do it for long, that's ok because Thanksgiving is just around the corner." It is important to first give yourself the opportunity to feel successful and to see if this goal is really in alignment with what you want.

I remember trying to get my baby daughter to go to sleep at night was really tough. I read every book written at the time about sleep training. Nothing worked; I was never able to let her cry it out or succeed with any of the other methods. It was incredibly stressful for both of us until I finally realized that I wanted to lie with her and read to her and listen to her breath until she fell asleep. I had to give myself permission to do it, instead of trying to do what I thought I should do because that is what worked for other people.

Now, just pause for a moment and think about what you want to create. What does it feel like? How would you feel if that was your reality? Getting very clear on what it is you want more of in your life helps focus your energy. After receiving a diagnosis like Hashimoto's, you basically have to start building your awareness and understanding of the condition, and at times you may feel you know more about it than your doctor.

Write a sentence with a very clear intention for you to achieve in the next three to six months. Write this intention in the present tense, and imagine the feeling you will embody when this is reality.

Here are a few examples:

- I eat in a way that gives me the energy I require to live well.
- I have an abundance of energy and I play with my children every day.
- I eat foods that make me feel healthy, vibrant, and strong.
- I have a morning ritual that creates stability in my body, I listen to my body's needs and support it.

Think about what specifically would solve a big problem for you. Now, write your own sentence stating a simple intention you would like to create in your life, one that will support your health and well-being. Remember to write it in the present tense.

Whatever your intention, spend time with it. Close your eyes and feel it. Every morning after your breath practice, repeat this intention three times mentally to yourself. Then feel grateful it has already happened. Spend time cultivating thoughts that align with your heart, and then see yourself in a year after consistently putting your health and wellness first. What are you doing, how do you feel, how do you look?

Just like I had to realize I actually wanted to stay with my daughter until she fell asleep, take stock. Notice if you embody a sense of joy when stating your intention. This feeling is as much what you want to cultivate as the words.

The more you build your awareness around your thoughts and feelings, the more aware you become of what things are energy sucks, what pull you down, or what things actually make you feel pure joy and connection.

Once you start to turn your attention to your energy, you will begin to notice periods throughout the day when your energy is higher than other times. A big contributor to your energy ups and downs may be connected to food.

Food

Food is one important component, and a great way we can choose to build or lower our energy on a daily basis. The fact is, the more toxins or low-grade food or drink you consume, the more energy your body will have to use to detoxify. Sometimes you may want to overindulge or eat a piece of chocolate cake, and that is totally fine as long as you do it with the understanding that you are exchanging part of your potential energy. It has been such a mindset shift for me to see food as potential energy.

Will this move me further toward my dreams or further away from them? At times, I may choose to have a glass of wine, for example, knowing I do have that savings account for a reason. Building awareness of the choices we constantly make helps us to be more conscious that greater potential is available and accessible right now. As soon as you make one better choice, then you are choosing to up your game.

As you start to move inflammation, it is important to maximize your ability to get good things into the body, i.e., oxygen and nutrients. Start in the gut, taking a good look at supporting your body with nutrition. Eliminate the things that are known to cause inflammation. You may not have to do so forever, but at the very least, give yourself an opportunity to know what foods potentially triggers an inflammatory response in your body and how much different you feel without them.

The lungs, the skin the intestines, the liver, and the kidneys are all organs of elimination. They support each other, working in the body to remove waste. If one of these organs is not functioning at optimal levels, it will begin to put stress on the others. For example, if you don't sweat very much, you may find you urinate more frequently than others, or that your breath is heavier. As I mentioned earlier everything is connected, and so it is as one organ is taxed, the other organs begin to take on the work load of the weaker organ. As we have discussed, it takes quite a bit of pain for us to pay attention, so one of your organs may have been working extra hard for a while now. Which is why it is important that you begin to notice what the body is communicating to you and how you can best support it with the things you eat and the things you don't. You can now see why statistically if you have one autoimmune condition it is likely you have another.

If you are dealing with anxiety, skin irritations, or any other discomfort that doesn't feel crippling, know it is a call to action. Your body is talking to you. It's doing exactly what it is supposed to do by communicating to you that something needs your attention.

Exercise

Exercise is another key component to this energy game. While exercise is essential to health, we must first evaluate our relationship to it. I had a yoga studio for years, and I got to experience firsthand this idea people have that if they are not pouring sweat and on the brink of total intensity, they don't feel they're being effective. If you go to a gym, you find all kinds of extremes: the music is turned way up, the air conditioning is turned way down (in the case of hot yoga reverse that), and people have this idea that it has to push them to their edge. Whatever happened to a nice, brisk walk in nature? As you are struggling with autoimmune disease, it is very important you realize that intensity is actually not where it is at. In fact, if after you exercise you feel like you need to rest or take a nap, this may be a sign that you don't have any energy reserves, and right now only light exercise or movement is going to help you. Have the courage to not do hard exercise for a while until you build up a bigger energy savings account, and then you can decide the best way to exercise for you. Short, relaxing walks in nature are a form of movement that will actually help to build your energy account, but notice what is too much. At first, it may be just a few minutes to relax the mind, but after a while you may notice you can extend it to 20 minutes or longer.

Yoga is a very effective method of integrating all aspects of ourselves, and so it is of huge value on this journey to wellness. Be sure that yoga is not just *asana* or the physical poses. Make the breath be the most important part of the class, let it guide you. If you are having a hard time keeping your breath steady, you are working outside your capacity and should back off a bit. Yoga teaches us about the depths of who we are and how to live in a space of authenticity, integrating all aspects of ourselves into this experience of life. It is not about being perfect, but about building the inner connection and wisdom as a guide to the divine.

So the work for you is to determine what you really want. If you haven't pondered this question, I recommend you spend a little time journaling. Don't skip over that. Do the work, write it down. What do I want? Don't worry about the hows or whys, just be honest and open with yourself. Give that little voice inside of you that has wild ideas the opportunity to speak and be heard. This is a big part of moving forward in a way that feels empowered.

A few years ago, while at an in-depth self-study class, I allowed that little voice inside of me to admit that I wanted to write a book. It was such a small idea, and at first the logical brain came in and was very quick to give me a list of all the reasons why I couldn't possibly do this. When this voice of "logic," otherwise known as self-doubt, shows up for you, have the courage to say today, you're going to go ahead and dream, and inhabit that feeling of achieving what you want. Continue to remain in this space, and soon the self-doubt begins to get lighter. Eventually you keep feeding the fire from your account, and you realize it is actually quite possible.

I have found that self-doubt usually comes from a place of lack. If this is your constant state, then you must go back to building your fire by pausing, resting, and gathering strength. It is not that you can't do something; it is literally a numbers game. Do you have the energy it will take to create the thing you want? If you don't but you try anyway, you will probably be stuck in this place of lack and failure because you are just burning your tinder. Let's be clear: it is not because you are not good enough or smart enough or capable enough, but because you lost before you started because you lacked the energy to make it happen.

Self-talk

I don't know what it is about negative self-talk. It's kind of crazy that we have such high expectations of ourselves and then get so mad when we don't follow through. Why don't we instead use the energy we waste on putting ourselves down toward trying to build ourselves up? Negative self-talk and shaming are truly an energy suck. They will, time and time again, deplete your reservoir. If you get stuck in this space of what I like to call *mind stuff*, it is toxic, and it takes energy to clear it out. As you read this, notice your thoughts: are you judging yourself? Maybe by saying, "See, I suck at everything, I am even constantly telling myself I can't do it, I'm not smart enough or good enough," you are still in the pattern. First, just see it, and then instead say, "I am good enough, I am smart enough, I support myself with kindness and I now have the tools I need to create the life of my dreams."

Recognize your dreams and hold space for them. Every day, make it a practice to see how much energy you can gather. Know that this is in service to your dreams and how you will show up in this world to live your purpose. Substitute actions that will build your energy for things that suck you dry. Here are some examples:

I am tired so I will watch TV.

Instead, lie down and rest, take a bath, or go for a short walk in nature.

I am feeling like I will never get it all done.

You won't, so give yourself a break and do the most important things. Try not to take yourself too seriously.

I am stressed, so I will go on Facebook as a distraction.

Put the phone down. Pause and breathe for two minutes.

I want chocolate cake (I want energy fast).

Instead, eat something that will create lasting energy, foods that will sustain. An example would be a smoothie that has fruit, protein powder or collagen, and some fat (an avocado). Or go and do a hot cold contrast therapy.

I want results now, so I go and get my butt kicked at cross fit.

Choose an exercise program that is gently building instead of just kicking your ass. It is much more likely you will stay consistent.

It takes courage to break habits and not choose instant gratification. The idea that you can have this now feels safer. I promise you it does not take a lot of time to start building your energy. In just a few short weeks, you will have dramatically changed your relationship to everything. Continue to build your energy until it feels like you might explode. Keep hearing the call to act and keep courageously holding space for the dream. Once you have recovered your energy and you are feeling stronger, then begin to take the steps you need to move forward. Reach out and get the help you need. Don't waste energy struggling with trying to figure out how to do things when you can get a coach to tell you exactly what to do. A coach will hold your hand and make the whole thing seem so much more accessible. This is such a great hack. Remember how precious the energy commodity is. If you don't know how to create what you want, then get a teacher. We should all have teachers, but also make sure your teacher has a teacher. This is a good indication that they will be able to guide you and hold space for you because somebody is doing that for them.

Passion for life is absolutely key to having a life filled with true joy, happiness, and freedom. Without passion, we are just surviving. You deserve more than that.

Building Energy
Spa

So we have discussed different ways that you can change your relationship to energy. Cultivating your relationship with energy and learning what it feels like to reside in a place of abundance will help you build your foundation of health. One great way to build energy is to take a shower with warm water for a few minutes, then turn it on cold for 30 seconds. Go back to warm for a few more minutes, and then cold for about a minute. Repeat as desired, building cold up to two minutes. This is great for flushing the circulatory system and building the mitochondria of each cell.

In yoga we have a breath practice called *Kapalabhati* that helps to detoxify and energize the body. I recommend you add this breath practice to your tool box. It is a great way to shift the energy in your body. Watch the video on the practice here: leahcarver.com

Chapter 5

Love and the Heart

*"Time is growing short. There are unexplored
adventures ahead of you. You can't live the rest of
your life worried about what other people think.
You were born worthy of love and belonging.
Courage and daring are coursing through you. You
were made to live and love with your whole heart.
It's time to show up and be seen."*
BRENÉ BROWN

The heart we all learned about in school is an organ that pumps blood through the body. With fresh blood comes a fresh supply of oxygen and nutrients, but it is so much more than this. We have the physical heart and the spiritual heart, our emotional heart and the energetic heart. I believe all aspects are connected and of course inter-related.

Our bodies are connected and electrically charged. We are made of the same elements as the stars. Our blood plasma has the same chemical make-up as the ocean, our bones the same minerals as the reefs. Two governing minerals of the nervous system are calcium and magnesium. When we are under stress, the body uses more of these minerals. Magnesium is also key to heart health. If the minerals are not being provided through diet at the same or at a greater rate than needed, the body will look to the bones to pull the minerals it needs.

We are a living, functioning microcosm of the universal macrocosm, a system far more complex than we can even begin to understand, and yet we can see the way the earth supports our natural functions. The more disconnected and further we get from the earth, the more difficult we find it to support our health.

As food becomes more and more processed, the minerals found in foods do not support or sustain us the way they used to, and so we have to look further or harder and become more discriminating about the source of our food. We move throughout our days, sometimes without stepping outside for any period of time other than walking into the grocery store or from the car to the house. Taking the time to immerse yourself into nature is a vital step in recovery. Sit in the garden and feel the effects of the sun's rays. Go to the beach for a walk or go for a hike in nature. Whatever source of nature that surrounds you, seek it out. Spend time there, let it nourish your soul. Connecting with nature reminds us we are just one small piece of something bigger, something spectacular.

So What Is Inflammation, Anyway?

Let's look at inflammation in the body as highway congestion. When you find yourself in a virtual parking lot on the highway, you have a few options: pull into a rest stop and take a break, find a way around the blockage, or just sit in the slow crawl of traffic inching your way along, hopeful that up ahead, progress is being made and soon the block will be cleared.

Your blood is like the highway, bringing oxygen and nutrients throughout the body and removing waste. If there is inflammation, you know there is a blockage. Traffic is stopped, meaning waste is not moving out very quickly and there is not much nutrition coming in. Sometimes this blockage is necessary – for example, when there is an infection, like strep throat. The lymphatic system stops clearing until the infection is destroyed. With autoimmune conditions, however, it is a different story. The body is having a misfire and reacting to things it may not normally react to. You find yourself getting more and more sensitive to foods, airborne allergies, etc. What can you do to get things moving more easily? How can you support your system? Specifically, you will have to look at stress, diet, exercise, and environmental exposure to toxins and other insults.

Imagine that up ahead, there has been an accident involving a semi, a landscape vehicle with a trailer, a car, and a motorcycle. I want you to think about your body's blood and lymph system like this. Which do you think creates the biggest blockage? What is the semi, and what is the motorcycle? How much effect will clearing the motorcycle have on the traffic flow vs clearing the semi? How much energy will it take? Sometimes, when we are feeling extremely run down, the only thing we have the ability to clear is the motorcycle, which will provide a little more movement and with it comes a bit more strength, and so we decide to clear from little to big. At other times, it's best to just go after the semi, knowing this will get the traffic flowing much sooner.

We must take the time to know where we are going to be the most effective. For my client Sarah, it was imperative she take it slow. She was feeling so exhausted that just a small amount of very focused effort made her feel better, whilst a big effort just completely exhausted her and sent her to bed for days, feeding her self-doubt and negative self-talk. Sarah had four children and found herself worrying about what kind impression she was making on them. She didn't want to appear sick to them, and so she would be exhausted every night when they finally went to sleep. She would fall asleep with them for a few hours, and then get up and do some of the dishes and prep for the next day before going back to bed. It seemed the only way she could get through her day was by using caffeine and sugar to give her pick-me-up and make her feel better. Sarah had to learn to be compassionate to herself. Trying to hide the way she was feeling was just making things worse. We changed her schedule slightly, she learned to ask for help, and she realized it was ok to give herself a little attention. She learned that by demonstrating self-care to her kids, she was giving them a blueprint for doing the same for themselves.

It can be difficult when trying to manage your autoimmune disease as well as your life. It is very hard to move forward, but much more difficult to stay where you are. You are motivated to change because the pain to stay still is so great. Right about the time of diagnosis, all of a sudden there is a recognition that life will not be much fun if you continue in the direction you are moving. The thing is, chances are you are not going to get totally better and unless you make some significant lifestyle changes they will get worse. The question is, are you ready to make these changes?

With Hashimoto's, we feel an increase in inflammation in our bodies. Depending on our own unique bodies, we may feel the inflammation differently. Pain or swelling of joints, a bloated tummy, fatigue, swollen ankles or feet, migraines, rashes, and stomach issues are just some of the ways inflammation shows up. Depending on our genetics, our environment, our conditioning, the food we eat, and our thoughts, we may find symptoms manifest themselves differently.

The Layers

Have you asked yourself recently how you're feeling? Oftentimes we reply with a list of symptoms. Can you relate? I think it's important to actually talk about the different layers of feeling states. On any given day, ask yourself how you are feeling emotionally, physically, energetically, mentally. You will soon notice that when you keep most of the answers in an unconscious place where you don't allow yourself to differentiate between these feeling states. But the more you recognize the difference, the greater your ability to shift, even if just in one area. For example, if today you wake up and the pain is greater than it has been for a while, you may feel frustrated, angry even. Energetically, you feel defeated and weak, and mentally you are overwhelmed. I have found that when we recognize the connection and separation, we can take action that will create some change immediately. Sit for a few minutes in inquiry and ask yourself how you feel on these different levels. In fact, just validating that you are actually sad beneath the frustration on a particular day may be difficult. Pull out your calendar and look at your schedule. How can you best support yourself today? Is there time for a bath before having to run out? When can you schedule some rest time? All of these actions will show you that you are the most important thing on your list. You are validating your own experience and seeing yourself with compassion.

Do you keep looking externally for someone to help or make it all better? Chances are, this is never going to happen. Why? Because it is not about anyone else, it is about your own relationship to yourself. If you learn to make time and treat yourself with love and compassion, you will shift the energetic heart and emotional heart, and when you shift these, you will be amazed at how other things start to change, too. Remember, it's all connected, so in order to get to a place of wellness, it is much more effective if we treat every layer of ourselves.

My client Jane had been working with these concepts for some time when she said to me, "I woke up this morning and I had more pain in my hands than I had experienced for a while. I sat with my discomfort and decided to take a bath, do some hand stretches in the water, and then run cold fusions over my hands. I can't tell you the relief I felt at having tools I knew would be helpful. It immediately changed the way I felt, I was happy because I knew I could help. I owned what I was feeling and took action to support it."

One of the hardest things to come to terms with for me after being diagnosed with autoimmune disease was this feeling of sadness or anger. At first, I felt like my body was failing me, and I couldn't understand why this was happening to me. I was angry. Of course, I soon realized my body wasn't failing me, I had been failing it. I hadn't been paying attention. Then I was sad. There was no way for me to know the big picture or to see that this disease would actually transform my life in ways I couldn't think possible. It made me look at everything, and the stronger my connection to my heart became, the more love seeped into every corner of my life.

I remember a client saying to me once "I just don't understand why this happened. I am so healthy. I eat well and exercise moderately." As we began to unpack her experience, it was quite evident that while she appeared to be taking good care of herself, she was actually fighting a war. While she ate relatively well, she was doing way too much.

The spiritual heart is another layer. Listening to your soul and knowing how to support that part of you often gets overlooked. At times, spiritual practices can feel like a chore because we forget the places they are filling in our lives. It does not matter which spiritual practice you choose. For me, it is yoga, meditation, and nature. For some, it's church and communion with others. All of these things fill a place within us, they help us to remember unconditional love and support. That we are one part of a whole.

When we sit quietly and give the deepest part of ourselves the opportunity to be heard, we are doing ourselves a great service. The Dalai Lama says "My religion is very simple. My religion is kindness." Often we are kind to others and forget to be kind to ourselves, to be gentle. It is not always choosing the easy path, but the one that will sustain the bigger, wiser, connected part of you.

Space Equals Potential

The amazing thing about these practices is they are working with the subtle body and so they build your ability to shift to a place of love and compassion. Space becomes available as soon as we stop using so much of the energy we were spending to push things away. Now you are beginning to see that the things we fear are not so big or dark and scary. This space will allow the process of detoxification to begin. Here is the thing with detoxification: as we start to move stuff out, it will all come to the surface. So it is important we have practices in place to stop us from suffering when we don't need to. Remember earlier, when I spoke about the body being a physical manifestation of your life? Like a living, breathing diary, it has lots of stored things it couldn't process at the time of the experience. As you start to detox, these stored items will come up, and your work is to not attach to them, but instead to see them, feel them, and let them move through you. Think of a storage unit you have had for decades. You haven't even stepped inside it in ten years. Do you really need any of the things in there? If you go to clear it out and look through every piece of paper and every picture, it will take you ages to get through, and then you will attach and want to keep lots of it. Sometimes it's easier to just not go through it. Get the few important things and just let go of the rest.

As your body begins to rid itself of its toxic load, you may notice changes in your physical pain as well. I have often heard clients say, "I haven't felt this pain in years." As we heal, our symptoms may reappear briefly, and they go in reverse order. It's not uncommon to be afraid when you feel a pain or a physical challenge you haven't felt in a while, and you remember when it was, at one point, crippling. But the pain doesn't stay, it just moves through on its way out.

As you let things go, you will find you feel lighter and easier about life. You start to feel more space and time for the things you like to do. You may realize that somewhere along the way you got this false belief that the point of your very existence was to make others around you happy, to be of service to them. Understand that if you don't take care of yourself, you can't take care of everyone else and to "take care" of the people in your life does not mean to try and make their life as easy as possible. As you learn to love yourself and honor the little wise voice inside you that pushes you to grow and to be bold, you will experience life at a level you never thought possible.

To think of an autoimmune condition as a purely physical disease is to turn your back on your heart. Autoimmune conditions are diseases of every level. For each of us, it started in a different place. Maybe it was triggered by emotion or stress or physical trauma – that is not what matters. What matters is that you are now ready to make the changes necessary to move you further toward what you truly desire, as opposed to what you think you should do. As it is a disease on every level, it can only be treated on every level. When you start building your connection to your heart and soul, it will help to give the fortification you need to be resilient and to make the changes that support the lifestyle you desire.

One of the things I love most about building awareness is that with these practices, you are actively shifting your practice to address what you are feeling. Grief or sadness is a common emotion after receiving a diagnosis of autoimmune disease. One of my favorite breath practices for working with sadness or a heaviness in the heart area is to imagine, on the inhale, breathing light into the heart area, and to let go of any feelings of heaviness, self-doubt or sadness on the exhale. Continue with this practice for two to five minutes or longer, if desired.

Self-care is no easy thing. It is often termed pampering, a term, if I am totally honest, that really annoys me. Self-care is not spoiling yourself, it is literally about turning our attention inward and just listening to what is needed. We have become so disconnected from our inner knowing, and until we can realize this is the foundation upon which our health as well as all our hopes and dreams are based, then we will constantly struggle. Don't think this means life will be perfect, it won't. But our structure will be sound.

If you are realizing your relationship with yourself is far from connected, start a practice of self-massage. I like to use coconut oil with a little of my favorite essential oil blend and just massage over my body, moving in the direction of the heart. I love to do this while my nutrient dense bath is running, so I can just climb in afterwards. One of my favorite baths is to run the water at about 104 degrees and soak for 10 minutes after which I run the cold water and put any joints or muscles under the cold water for about 30 seconds. You can repeat this as desired. The contrast in temperature causes a clearing out of toxins and an increase in nutrient rich blood flowing through the body. It is not indulgent to care for this body. Think about it for a moment: What is the one thing we have on the day we are born that we still have on the day we die? This body, this vessel! Why would you not take the time to care for it and check in make sure it is functioning at optimal levels? Right now, you may feel like you are going to have to invest more time because for so long you have neglected yourself, but sometime in the future, you will see this practice of life propels you through your days, your weeks, and your years. It means you are not building castles in the sand, but instead you are building your legacy. It really allows you to be who you are.

As you go through your day, take a few moments whenever possible to walk outside. Include nature in your day, it is such a source of power and remembrance, connecting us back to our bodies and igniting the recognition that life is so much bigger than us and even the smallest ant has purpose. As you cook dinner for yourself or your family, infuse your cooking with fresh herbs from your herb garden. If you don't have an herb garden, just start small with a few small potted plants. It is amazing to breathe in the essence of the herbs as you prepare them for cooking.

Chapter 6

Wisdom

"The primary cause of unhappiness is never the situation, but your thoughts about it."
ECKHART TOLLE

ave you ever had an experience of just knowing something was right for you and then actually trusting that knowing? That is the voice of wisdom. It resides in each of us, but we have learned not to trust it, not to listen.

I remember when I was about 12, struggling to understand why people had different religious beliefs and how people "knew" that the religion they practiced was the right one. I talked to my mother about it. I was interested, but I was also aware it could be a sticky subject. For me, I found at an early age that the truth is what you believe in your heart. If what you believe is not working for you, then change your truth. Question why or how this became your truth.

69

I remember being pregnant and thinking, "Wow, everyone is pregnant!" It wasn't true; there were not an unusual number of pregnancies or births that year, it was just that I was looking for confirmation of my reality all around me. You see no other truth but that which you believe matters. That's why, in Buddhism, one of the first thing they ask you to do is break down all of your belief systems. It's difficult to do – your beliefs are formed at an age where you don't realize it's a belief system and not just facts.

What does this have to do with you and your Hashimoto's? Have you taken any time to think about what you believe about this autoimmune disease? Grab your journal and ask yourself why you think you got an autoimmune condition. Try not to answer from the head, but ask your heart, and answer from there. Remember to be kind to yourself. Don't judge what you have written. It may not even be true, and yet there may be something in it that needs a little more unpacking. Right now, you are just starting to ask the questions and building a relationship with what you are feeling.

Now ask yourself, "Do I believe I can regain my health?"

It is vitally important that you believe this is possible. But just because I say it is important doesn't mean you can automatically believe it. Don't be too quick to pretend you believe it is possible. Take a moment and feel it. Say it: "I can regain my health." Now upgrade it to: "I am healthy and feel gratitude."

Make a note, write down how healthy feels to you.

Your support team, your community, the people you talk to and the books you read, the movies you watch – all of it is precious and will either move you toward your goal of a healthy, happy, fulfilling life, or further from it.

Is there a part of you, an inner voice, who has been talking to you for a while? Can you take a moment and give that part of you the opportunity to be heard? Write a letter to yourself from the deepest, wisest part of you. As often as possible, learn to hear this voice and give her the opportunity to speak. I recommend doing this practice daily. For three to five minutes in the morning, seek council from this deep source of wisdom and knowing within you. Be bold and allow this relationship to blossom.

It's time in the journey to get a little deeper, to look more at the internal workings of your mind. Your scariest truth: Can you hear it? Can you speak it? What do you think is your greatest fear? Maybe it is the fear of failure, but beneath that you may find it is actually the fear of your light. Rip it up and throw it away if it feels too big just yet, but begin to give a voice to that part of you that has been quiet for so long. Own your inner conflict, we all have it. Even those of us who seem to have it all figured out.

Do the work of getting to know yourself. Just because you hear and speak some of these deep worries, fears, or dreams does not mean they are true. But you must give them a voice to see if it resonates with what you believe, and then to know whether that belief serves your greater good. If it doesn't, replace it with one that does. It can feel a little difficult at first, but will help you to energetically shift and let go of thoughts you have been carrying around that don't serve you – in fact, they just eat up your energy. You don't get to choose everything that happens to you in life, but remember you do get to choose how you show up, what your response is like, and how you direct the flow. Are you willing to look?

Is what you are doing right now working for you (hint: obviously not)? And if not, why are you so attached to it? This is where a good sense of wonder can really come in handy. Wonder why, if it is not working, it seems easier. Wonder why, if we are living in a state of physical, mental, emotional pain, we are afraid to make changes. Wonder. Wonder, and wonder some more. Begin to ask yourself these questions.

In autoimmune disease, the body has literally become confused about where the "enemy" is. When we are under chronic stress, be it physical, mental, or emotional, there comes a breakdown of proper function. Our bodies are telling us we need to limit the amount of information coming in, give it some time to process the things it is storing. This is why pausing, resting, and then accessing the heart and inner awareness works. Until we do these things, it will be hard to interrupt the pattern.

Often throughout this life it seems we are just waiting for things to happen to us. So much of the time, we give our power away. I have been surrounded by strong women all of my life. I have some truly amazing and inspiring people I can turn to for help or advice, but in a way, I hid behind these people like a child flirting with someone from behind the folds of their mother's skirt. I wanted to be seen, and yet I was scared to go it alone. When I really started to struggle with Hashimoto's, it was the first time that I began deciding what would be best for me without first factoring in all the people I loved and cared about into the equation. I had to set boundaries for myself, and because of these boundaries, I was able to own my own strength. At a time when I felt the weakest, I found a different kind of strength.

Hashimoto's totally interrupted the pattern of my life and if I'm being totally honest, it needed a little interruption. Now of course it could have gone the other way, but thankfully for me, I had been prepping for this work for years. All the knowledge and passion I had directed at helping other people I was now able to put it into a practice for me. It was the push I needed to trust my inner knowing and take action.

Is it luck that things are good, or can you create and craft your own reality? I have a friend who is a musician and have heard him say how frustrating it can be when people say, "Oh you are so talented," like he just woke up one day and could play and sing music. The truth is that most people who excel at things have a little raw talent, but beneath that they have the dedication to practice every day. They know this is what they want to spend their time doing. It isn't easy, but they are willing to work at it. They understand that to be great at what they do, they have to practice. Without practice, they will never reach their potential.

Daily practice can be no easy thing, especially when it comes from a place of rigidity. Not only do you have to make the time and put it above all things, but it takes having the resiliency to show up without attachment to the results. No excuses. Developing your inner awareness, your ability to hear the call, and to act is one of the greatest ways to develop personal power. When we act in alignment with our inner authenticity, we are unstoppable. That doesn't mean it will be easy, but we are more resilient and we are much more willing to keep trying.

Living in this day and age is amazing and challenging. We have instant gratification at our fingertips. It is easy to get distracted from the big picture and to get pulled into some great or not-so-great amusement. There can be too many options, too many recommendations of how best to do it, too many ways to change track. Who would think this would be a problem? For us it is usually not a lack of information, but rather too much. This is where developing inner knowing can be so helpful. We become aware of our tendencies. Some will get paralyzed by just gathering information, others will be off trying harder, and still others will be spending as much time as possible in social situations avoiding the issue.

Gratitude is the quality of being thankful, or a readiness to show appreciation for and to return kindness. The second part of the definition is especially true in regard to the attitude we want to develop with our Hashimoto's. You want to cultivate a readiness to show appreciation for the message the body is giving you and to return with kindness. You can change the belief that this is bad and your body is failing you to gratitude for the wake-up call, and in response, be willing to be kind to yourself, be willing to care for yourself. Gratitude that we have been given a reminder of what is truly important. Gratitude that more and more information is being made available. Thank goodness for the technological age, because it helps get the information out to us faster. You are being called to be bold, to step up and own your disease. No more excuses, they don't matter and they won't get you better.

Autoimmune disease can seem scary and overwhelming. There are no quick solutions or easy answers for most of us. If we ignore it, it accelerates, and if we want to change it, we have to become our own advocates, we have to search out the best doctors, we have to keep throwing mud at the wall and that takes energy when we don't have any. The practices and tools in this book are here to support you, not to replace sound medical advice but to empower you day by day. Unfortunately, or maybe it is fortunately, we can't do things the way we used to or the ways others do them, we have to be more diligent. If you want to change the way this disease is ransacking your life, then you must draw it in close. You cannot push it away. No amount of wishing it was different will get you there. Is now the time? If it's not, ask yourself why this isn't the most important thing in the world right now.

When we connect with our truth, we stop looking for society to dictate the best way of living for us, and we are able to recognize where we are out of alignment. The sickness resides in the place of not listening to the call of our hearts, of our dreams, and our desires. Instead, we're letting fear hold us back and keep us small. We must become advocates of our own health and of our children's. This is the perfect opportunity to remember that life will ebb and flow. At times it will be difficult and feel like it takes all of you to get through it, but at others you can recognize the beauty of the cliff you just scaled or the magnificent blessings that surround you. These practices help you recognize all the beauty that is available to you, even in the struggle, and so they keep you steadfast on your path.

We are at war with an invisible enemy and our bodies, our so very wise bodies, are telling us to pay attention. Dig deep. Is what you are doing now truly working for you? If it's not, I can promise you without a doubt that it will not get better without you owning it and changing it. Be a warrior for change. I know right now that may feel overwhelming – you are exhausted and maybe depressed – but once you start to feel better, you will want to take on the world. Right now, your energy is low and you have little capacity to create big change. But your inner voice is calling you, it is begging you. As you notice the shift from exhaustion to empowerment, you will also become aware of how good it feels to feel good! Your dreams will take up residence once again, and you will be unwilling to go back.

The Three Questions is a children's book I have read many times to my kids. In it, a wise turtle answers a boy's three questions: What is the most important time? Who is the most important one? What is the most important thing to do?

The only important time is now. The most important one is the one in front of you. The most important thing is to do good. As you read these chapters, know the most important time is now, the most important person is yourself, and the most important thing to do is to take care of yourself so that you can then fulfill your destiny, have access to your power, and show up in a way that is your soul's authentic expression. Every morning, just take a few minutes to yourself to check in and write down your musings.

If you are having a difficult time integrating your inner and outer realities, then I suggest adding a practice of body brushing. The skin is part of the nervous system. In fact, I have heard it called the nervous system turned inside out. One of the main functions of the skin is communication. It is in direct relationship with the brain, telling it if something is too hot or cold, or pressure is too hard or too light. We can use this relationship to send soothing messages to the brain.

Think about the skin in this sense. Have you ever had a massage and while you are trying to relax, you are absolutely freezing and so you are tensing all your muscles? It's not very enjoyable is it? This is why in spas it is a common practice to have bed warmers, creating a conducive environment for relaxation. It is a common practice for people with anxiety disorders or insomnia to sleep with a heavy duvet because it helps calm the nervous system.

Body brushing has many effects, but this is one of the most exciting: it works directly with the skin, and since the skin shares nerve pathways with many of the organs of the body and has a direct connection to the brain, it can be a very effective practice. I also love that you can work to speed up the flow of lymph which is directly related to the removal of waste. Body brushing is energizing, so make sure you only do it in the morning.

Chapter 7

Evolve

"Meditation moves the brain in the direction of rest and focus. Thus, learning to still your mind is not only a vital link to inspiration and an abiding sense of peace but also an incomparable method for increasing your capacity to solve real-life issues, increase insight, and help your brain assimilate all the random bits of information that it rarely has time to process. Meditation is an indispensable tool that improves memory, sharpens intellect, increases your ability to stress, and even helps you to process negative emotions such as grief, anger, and fear."

ROD STRYKER, *THE 4 DESIRES*

After my diagnosis of Hashimoto's, the natural question was: Why? I think this is our response to most negative things that happen to us, right? Why me, why now?

Why is this so hard? I now know without a doubt that getting Hashimoto's has been in service of my growth and I wouldn't change it for the world, but at the time, I wondered what I did to deserve it. Why was it so hard for me when I had tried "to be good" and do the right thing?

More than ever before, I have been asked to show up in a way that feels uncomfortable and at times downright dark, and yet I can honestly say I feel more powerful than ever. I have greater access to my dreams, I know my heart, and I smile kindly upon my challenges. So, no, I'm not perfect, and I am not totally healed. Yes, I still have days that are tough, but I see them for what they are: a choice! What do I choose today: to be stuck or to grow?

I have tools I can use to facilitate energetic change in my body. If I'm not using them, then I have to ask what I am getting out of where I am residing. There is a part of you, a subconscious part that is creating the same situation in different forms over and over again. When have you had enough? When is it time to recognize it for what it is, to smile gently in reflection, and to choose a different, unfamiliar path? "When?" has become my new question. When am I going to act in accordance with my soul? When am I going to pay attention to this? When will I choose discomfort in the present to evolve the cycle? My answer is always, "Now."

I have found myself in the place I never expected. All the soul searching I had done before was not getting me the answers I needed. It felt elusive, and I struggled. Almost everything I did came from a place of "I should." I have realized I had stopped wanting to do a lot of things that previously felt fun or interesting. Everything just became effort. I felt my world getting smaller and smaller. As I went through this process, however, I felt my energy begin to increase. In a way that felt steady and yet inspired, I could once again engage in life the way I wanted. I stopped being angry and frustrated because I was feeling exhausted or overwhelmed. My practice began to deepen, and once again I began to meditate.

Try to understand, my yoga practice was and is such an important part of my life, but for a while I had to change it. That is the beauty of it. For so many, we equate *asana* with yoga, and it simply is not. In fact, I do very little *asana* these days, though I'm sure there will be days where I do more. I needed to take time every day to make sure I was doing practices that were gentle and were going to leave me feeling steadier and more nurtured than I had before. I didn't judge myself while doing practices that reminded me how to soften.

The stories we tell and the judgments we usually pass on ourselves in answer to the "why" question are just that, stories, and they can be a distraction. One of the first steps to wellness is to recognize the problem. That is why we use the Big Pause to identify the thoughts behind the problem. Hashimoto's is not the problem, the problem is our body is communicating to us and we may not be listening or willing to make the changes it requires to support us. As long as we push the problem away, we can make no space for growth. We search for the best doctor, and then don't do what they tell us to do. We wish for them to fix it, but they can only help – the rest is on us. Owning the problem, however, means we are open to guidance. We can look to our inner teacher, doctor, or coach to assist us in recognizing our patterns and keeping us accountable to our dreams. They will direct us on the path to wellness, but we must show up.

Seeing yourself as a part of a greater whole can be incredibly powerful. Connection is defined as a relationship in which a person, thing, or idea is linked or associated with something else. It is one of the things we have forgotten, and yet our soul searches for it. If you look at our medical system, for example, you will see some major flaws, but one of the worst in the case of autoimmune disease is the specialist.

One of my clients, Liz, had gone to her doctor and complained of fatigue and struggling to get out of bed, a feeling of overwhelm and sadness. The doctor referred her to a psychiatrist, and she was put on an antidepressant. You see, so frequently the symptoms are treated, but not the whole person. A specialist is usually just going to treat you within the scope of their practice instead of working with the entire body to piece together all of the parts. Thank goodness functional medicine is on the rise, and hopefully we will see more and more access to functional medicine doctors. When my mother first came to America as a health and beauty practitioner, she was told she would have to choose between getting a cosmetology license and a massage license. She had never done hair in her life, and so she chose initially to just do massage. She couldn't understand, though, how you could possibly treat one part of the body without treating the whole. This propelled her forward with her life's work to teach traditional spa treatments as the therapies they were designed to be.

The skin is the mirror organ of the body, so how can you be an effective esthetician without taking the health of the body into account? Years ago, when I worked at a large spa, I had a VIP press client in. She asked me which facial would be the best to get her skin looking healthy and vibrant, and I recommended she actually have a seaweed wrap. The treatment involved body brushing, an essential oil application, and a very rich mineral seaweed. The physical theory behind the service was to begin moving the lymphatic system with the body brushing, continue to support the movement of waste with a very specific oil application, and then to apply seaweed, a food source, to feed the body through the skin. On an emotional level, the aromas of the essential oils created a relaxation state, you felt nurtured and could relax. The nervous system was stimulated by the body brushing, the gentle rocking movements and the smooth application. This was an experience that would treat you at every level of your being.

As you learn how to work with the intelligence of the physical body, you gain greater insight and access into the soul. The body is in constant relationship with your soul. It will act as a catalyst, pushing you constantly to grow. There are many, many layers to these complex human spiritual beings that we are, and it's important to know that each and every layer has something to offer. Evolution is not about elevating us above our humanness and neglecting this physical body, but more about pulling it in, holding it with tender loving arms. The body is wise, listen to the depths of what it is saying, be discerning and it will guide you towards your heart. As you begin to value what your body is communicating to you (as opposed to just wishing it would be different or pushing it away), you will create a new, connected relationship with yourself that is based on love and respect.

Connection is a universal theme, but sometimes we can't see how everything, including ourselves, is connected. Let's take trees, for example. Trees come from seeds, break through the dirt floor, and sprout up. Growing towards the sun, they are in constant communication with the environment around them. They are a part of something, rooted, growing, and developing branches and flowers. More than likely, they will weather a few storms and their branches will break, but hopefully, their roots are strong. Branches will grow back, they will produce seeds, and continue the reproductive cycle. Trees are a source of many things: oxygen, shelter, and food, just to name a few. Without trees, I don't know that we could exist.

The examples from nature that everything is connected are plentiful, from plants to insects. Everything is living and breathing and working within a system. Our bodies are like their own unique universe. We are the microcosm and are in relationship with the universe at large, the macrocosm. The first step to tending to our earth is to tend to ourselves.

Part of our human nature makes us focus externally. Maybe it is conditioning, or maybe it is the nature of our being. In order to do the big stuff you came here to do, it is vital to value yourself, to be respectful of your body. But also take the time to realize and walk in awareness of the relationship you are in with nature and the earth. Bathe in the natural waters around you, breathe in the clean mountain air, frolic in the meadow again as you did as a child. Yes, I said frolic – how long has it been since you did that? This connection is a great source of energy for us. It will feed us and sustain us.

We live in a sick world. Thyroid specialist Isabella Wentz says, "Somewhere between 13.5 percent and 27 percent of the general population in the US has thyroid antibodies, which indicates that they have Hashimoto's."

People are suffering, and I believe whole heartedly it is a call to action. Our bodies are saying, "Don't get distracted, changes need to be made." We must heal ourselves and heal the world. We must own this epidemic and work evolve it. Our planet is sick. We must understand that the relationship between humans and our planet is symbiotic. We are dependent upon the Earth to provide our sustenance, our oxygen, and our water, and she is dependent upon us to be good stewards of the planet. Our life and legacy depend upon it. Earth is the macrocosm, and we are the microcosm reflecting back. To live in harmony with it means to not always make the easy choice, but to do the work to make the necessary changes.

Perspective

I had a friend tell me about a car accident she was in recently. Her story about how the accident occurred was completely different than the other driver's. Now there could be several reasons for this, but one of them was that the other driver just didn't want to accept responsibility, so they chose to see what happened very differently, even believing, I'm sure, the story themselves. Other people who had witnessed the accident had pulled over and so were able to confirm the story my friend told. I don't necessarily think that the woman who caused the accident was consciously lying. I am sure that she just saw a reality that would confirm what she wanted to believe and chose that instead. In fact, I have read that when under stress, we stop filtering the negative and only look for positive, reassuring information, which may be why we make some pretty silly decisions from stress and why clever sales people can make you feel extreme stress and fear so you buy their products.

It is important as we grow and evolve that we take the opportunity to continue to question our perspective. It is only when we keep our minds open to the idea that there may be another way we are not able to see that we remain open to change. Keeping an open mind is easier said than done, right? After all, most of us are operating in a chronic stress state that keeps the mind from being open. This is why having practices that build your steadiness also helps expand your perspective. All of a sudden, you find yourself noticing a path you never saw before. It can feel a little like magic, and yet it is simply giving yourself a broader base so the gentle wind doesn't just blow you over. The more time we invest in building our inner awareness and power through practices like breath work, meditation, and introspection, the greater ability we will have to show up in the world the way we want to.

I have suggested several practices to you by now, but I want to be clear that you are not *supposed* to be doing anything. The only thing I ask is that you try each of the practices for seven days so you can fully evaluate if they are working for you or not. Give them a chance to work their magic. I think you will be amazed at the amount of energy these very simple practices can add to your life. While I did go a little bit into diet and exercise, it is not my main focus of this book. There are some amazing books on protocols written by some incredible people out there. It was my experience that all that knowledge did me absolutely no good because I couldn't take action. I was crippled by willpower fatigue, and so the purpose of this book is to build your willpower back up, to fill your energy tank so that you can make powerful, life-changing choices in a way that feels good, reconnects you to your dreams and desires, and allows you to see your potential.

Meditation

After all the prep work you have done, now it is time to start a meditation practice. If you have never done mediation before, just recall how you feel when you do something you enjoy. There is an ease to it, and a lightness. Meditation helps you to learn how to get yourself to that place, a place of softness and ease that helps you become more expansive. As you practice regularly, you will see the subtle shift of consciousness take up residence in your life.

Begin with a balanced breath practice, a one-to-one count, inhale and exhale. Continue to follow your breath as your mind and body become more quiet or relaxed. Continue to relax. Relax your shoulders, your jaw. Allow the breath to relax as the mind gets quiet. Put your awareness behind the navel in the belly. Feel the gentle movement of the breath. Relax the breath after a few minutes, but if you notice your mind gets busier, i.e., thoughts of grocery shopping, the day ahead, etc., then start the breath again, counting the length of inhale and the length of exhale. Don't worry about doing it right, the more time you spend doing this the more comfortable you will get. Just like anything else, don't expect yourself to be an expert; whatever your experience is, it's perfect. Begin with 10 minutes. If this feels too hard, then shorten the practice. Remember, it is a feeling of gentleness, softening, and steadiness we are looking to cultivate. This is a key part of your journey.

Meditation and breath work will help you recognize early "warning signs" or messages from the body. The more attuned you can become, the more you will be able to take actions that support continuing a sense of ease in your life. For a guided meditation, you can look on my website leahcarver.com

Chapter 8

Obstacles

Good news! You made it to Chapter 8 and through all the steps! I have written this chapter and called it "Obstacles" because, let's face it, the reason you are reading this book is because you need help. Things will always come up and try to get in the way. In each chapter, I have given you at least one practice. I call it a practice because you are practicing to build a relationship with your inner self and to interpret the messages your body is relaying to you. You should have no expectation of doing this all perfectly straight away.

Through managing my Hashimoto's, I realized the amount of pressure I would sometimes put on myself to be able to do things that I had no previous experience with. One of my biggest lessons through this is if you have the information and are still struggling to take the actions you need to take, then get a teacher or coach. Think about this. For most of our adolescent life, we had parents, teachers at school, athletic coaches – any time we started a new hobby, there was someone there to teach us at least the basics. At some point, you get a job, a house, and have a child or two – and it is at this point when we usually stop having a teacher. We have all kinds of new responsibilities, but no teacher or coach. And yet somehow we just expect we should know how to do these things. And this is the kicker: we get very frustrated and feel guilty when we screw up. Why? At what point do we start to have these crazy expectations of ourselves?

I have found, in working with my clients over the years, that until you value yourself, until you make the time to care for yourself, you will always be short on time. Yes, you heard that right! You have to invest time, actually taking time out of your day, in order to make time. I fought this for a long while. Obviously, time is not actually created, but when you have built a solid foundational practice like the one in this book, you have learned the power of listening to your soul. All kinds of things that will distract you from yourself will fall away. As they do, you find more space and time to do the things in alignment with you. Trust me and trust the process. If you had told me a few years ago I would have the energy to be doing what I am doing now, I would have laughed. I was so tired that I was not functioning well at all.

It is incredible how much time we lose in the cracks, just mindlessly scanning Facebook or watching TV. I get that you feel too tired to do anything else, but if you practice the actions in this book, you will see what I mean. You will notice that you get much more done in a day, and you feel better doing it.

But watch out for the tendency to try too hard or overdo it. Remember to be kind to yourself. Don't get upset with yourself if you are not doing what you are "supposed" to be doing. If it feels like work, then you will not do it. If that is the case and you are feeling this as a to-do list, then just stick to the basics. For example, simply take a nutrient-filled bath every day, try not to make it too hot, but enjoyable. Once you notice a shift in how you are feeling, then add another practice. Give each practice time to sink in.

There will be days when you forget the importance of this practice. Those days are there to remind you. Do not see them as failures, just lessons. Notice the difference in the way you navigate your day when you have your practice in place versus the days you don't.

Remember the more good energy you can put into your body, the less your body will have work and burn energy to remove toxins. Energy is the most important commodity! On days where you know you will need to put more energy out – for example, your child's birthday is coming up, she is having a slumber party and you know this will be exhausting for you – start to build your energy by resting more in the days leading up to the party.

Balance your energy checkbook every day. Once you start to feel a little more energy, you get excited and can overdo it. Remember, you have empty coffers to fill before you feel the excess. Store it up and see what you can do. When stuff comes up, and it will, Pause, rest, build, connect, and listen before you take action. Run a bath and do your practice. It's that simple –not to be confused with easy. Show up for yourself daily, whether you are feeling good or not so good. No excuses. Just do the practice without attachment to the result, do the practice. If you find yourself struggling, reach out and get the help you need.

Conclusion

One of the most important things to remember on this journey is that while at times it feels isolating and difficult, know you are not alone. In fact, it is estimated that 27 percent of the population is with you. Does that make you feel better? Me neither, because if in fact you were alone, it would mean we don't really have a crisis on our hands. And I mean "us" as a community and as a collective. Unfortunately, we do! It is not a fluke, and it is happening to women everywhere. We have to evolve this epidemic because if we don't, what does that mean for our children and their children?

The answers provided in this book come from the ancients. They represent age-old advice and practices that have stood the test of time. They are here to remind you that you are so much more complex than anyone can understand. Beneath it all, you are energy, you are the stars and the sea. What you surround yourself with on a daily basis, be it internal or external, defines that energy. Choose wisely!

There is purpose in Hashimoto's, and I believe it is to wake us up. It is a call to action. To remind us we are one part of a greater whole, and that all parts matter. As we see the breakdown of the food industry, the medical industry, and society, we are being called to see there is a different, better way. If we come together and evolve, we can create more than we have ever dreamed possible. The status quo will not work for us anymore. We must stand up and use our voices. It is so important that we recognize our self-worth, our individual purpose, and our collective purpose.

Recently I saw *Wonder Woman* in the movie theater. At the end of the movie, it all comes down to one moment. It is apparent that there is darkness in the world, and it is strong. It can be a force to be reckoned with, but there is also light, and when you chose light, you realize it is so much stronger than the dark. Just a small candle will light up a room.

It is my hope that you remember the light you are. That you feel the fire burning within and that you now have the tools to keep it burning strong. Remember, I am available if you need support.

I know there is a place inside you that burns bright. Let that brightness shine and help light others up. It may not be easy at times, but every superhero has her tools, use them wisely. Be open to reevaluating everything. Work on letting go of ideas that haven't served you. Now is your time. Live your purpose, and love well!

Acknowledgments

Allen, my loving husband, for always being in support of my dreams and reminding me to slow down and remember the beauty all around me.

My daughters, Ella and Charlotte, for inspiring me to be bold and the best version of myself.

Sara, my sister and friend, who has been on this journey with me since birth. Thanks for always being in it with me.

My mother, for teaching me to be true to my heart.

My father, for loving me unconditionally.

My brother, for making me tough and making me laugh.

My students and clients, who ask the questions and do the work.

Angela Lauria, for giving me courage to own my truth.

Maggie McReynolds, for your encouragement.

Dr. Gabrielle Knaus, for always supporting me and problem-solving with me.

Kim Marrone, for putting me on the path back to wellness.

My teacher, YogaRupa Rod Stryker: your wisdom and teachings have inspired me and taught me so much. Thank you for holding space and the deep sense of comfort.

Lani - for inspiring love in the truest sense.

To my communities and my people – my dear friends and family – I feel so blessed.

To the Morgan James Publishing team: Special thanks to David Hancock, CEO & Founder for believing in me and my message. To my Author Relations Manager, Bonnie Rauch, thanks for making the process seamless and easy. Many more thanks to everyone else, but especially Jim Howard, Bethany Marshall, and Nickcole Watkins.

About the Author

Leah Carver is an author, founder of the Claim Your Health, Claim Your Life movement, a successful entrepreneur, and spa wellness coach. She is a certified spa therapist and yoga teacher who has been working for the last 20 years to help her clients on a path to health and happiness. Leah found out during her own health challenges 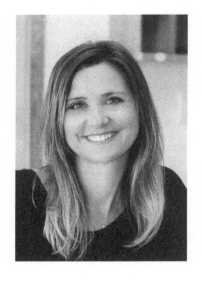 sometimes we may know what to do, but struggle to actually do it. She learned firsthand after being diagnosed with Hashimoto's how powerful yoga and spa therapy can be in your recovery. She used these tools daily to bring her body back to balance. Leah is teaching people to change their perspective and see their potential from a different angle.

Leah has been taught by some of the most amazing teachers within the spa and yoga industries. She holds an ASTECC certification for Spa Therapies from Anne Bramham, and studied Lymphatic drainage under Hildegard Wittlinger of The Dr. Vodder School. While she has studied many traditions of yoga, Leah now considers herself lucky to be the student of Rod Stryker and ParaYoga. She has owned both a spa and yoga studio. Leah has traveled across the United States teaching at spas. Some of the spas Leah has taught at are Spa Montage and Canyon Ranch. Leah is excited to take the ancient teachings of spa therapy to the public. She teaches retreats, coaching programs, and VIP spa days.

Leah lives in Jupiter, FL on a small bonsai farm with her husband, her two daughters, her dog, cat, chickens, and the occasional chaos.

Thank You

Hey, thanks for reading *Undoing Hashimoto's*! This is just the beginning of your journey on the path to wellness and managing your symptoms of Hashimoto's, but it is my hope for you that the book and the practices contained within have given you the stability and rock-solid foundation you need to support the lifestyle changes you want to make from a place of power and certainty. There is nothing like being in pain and feeling like you don't know what to do to help yourself.

As a thank you to readers to this book, I've created a video of my personal five favorite spa hacks. You can find it here: undoing.leahcarver.com

"Claim Your Health, Claim Your Life."

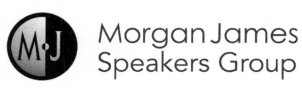

Morgan James
Speakers Group

↗ www.TheMorganJamesSpeakersGroup.com

We connect Morgan James published
authors with live and online events
and audiences who will benefit
from their expertise.

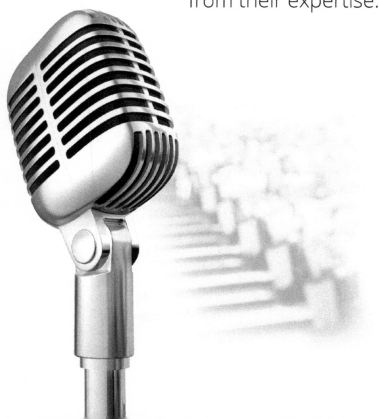

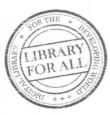